Diabetic Sweet Tooth Cookbook

Mary Jane Finsand

Foreword by James D. Healy, M.D., F.A.A.P.

Sterling Publishing Co., Inc. New York

Edited by Laurel Ornitz
Recipe consultant: Carol Tiffany

Library of Congress Cataloging-in-Publication Data

Finsand, Mary Jane
   Diabetic sweet tooth cookbook / Mary Jane Finsand ; foreword by
James D. Healy.
   p.   cm.
   Includes index.
   ISBN 0-8069-8530-5
   1. Diabetes—Diet therapy—Recipes.   2. Desserts.   I. Title.
RC662.F5673   1993
641.8′6—dc20   92-31090
                                              CIP

10 9 8 7 6 5 4

Published by Sterling Publishing Company, Inc.
387 Park Avenue South, New York, N.Y. 10016
© 1993 by Mary Jane Finsand
Distributed in Canada by Sterling Publishing
% Canadian Manda Group, P.O. Box 920, Station U
Toronto, Ontario, Canada M8Z 5P9
Distributed in Great Britain and Europe by Cassell PLC
Villiers House, 41/47 Strand, London WC2N 5JE, England
Distributed in Australia by Capricorn Link Ltd.
P.O. Box 665, Lane Cove, NSW 2066
Manufactured in the United States of America

Sterling ISBN 0-8069-8530-5

Contents

Foreword

In *Diabetic Sweet Tooth Cookbook*, Mary Jane Finsand has created recipes for scrumptious desserts using many of the newest sugar replacements. These desserts allow diabetics and other people on restricted diets to enjoy "sweets" occasionally. Users of Mary Jane's other diabetic cookbooks know that diabetics can eat a wide variety of delicious foods and still follow their doctor's recommendations.

Each recipe includes calories and food exchanges for each serving. This completeness allows diabetics to regulate food intake within a medically prescribed diet while eating a wide variety of foods. Please share this cookbook with your own doctor, pharmacy, hospital dietician, and diabetic organization. I am confident that they will confirm my high recommendation.

James D. Healy, M.D., F.A.A.P.

A Note from Covenant Medical Center

Diabetic Sweet Tooth Cookbook shows you safe ways to have your cake and diabetes, too! This resource can help people with diabetes add flavor, sweetness, and variety to their diet while continuing to control their blood-glucose levels.

We encourage patients at the Diabetes Health Center at Covenant Medical Center to select cookbooks that have been written by a credible author and include nutritional analysis, American Diabetes Association exchanges, and tested recipes. We have found that this book as well as other cookbooks by Mary Jane Finsand meet these criteria.

Our patients are reminded that these "sweet" items need to be substituted into the diabetic meal plan. Unfortunately, you cannot always have your cake and your bread, too.

We also recommend self-blood-glucose monitoring to discover what effects diet changes will have on your blood-glucose levels. If you do not have a diabetes meal plan appropriate for your lifestyle, we encourage you to contact a registered dietician.

Mary Steffensmeier, R.D.
Lynette Gersema, R.N.
Covenant Medical Center
Waterloo, Iowa

Introduction

People on any diet often feel that food falls into two categories: good and bad. And of all the bad foods, none are considered worse than desserts. Desserts normally are thought of as a nonessential luxury, eaten purely for pleasure. No wonder we all feel so guilty eating a dessert.

But perhaps it is time to rethink our attitudes. A sweet after a meal may give us the psychological edge we need to continue eating healthy meals and stay on our prescribed diet.

A dessert can be nothing other than fresh fruit. Not only is fruit tasty and refreshing, but it is low in calories, cholesterol, and fat, and it contains plenty of vitamins, minerals, and fibre. In addition, there are many sweeteners on the market that can be used in recipes to keep the calories and exchanges down to a minimum.

In this cookbook, I have tried to create recipes that are healthy and low in calories and exchanges but score high in taste. I hope you enjoy them. I also hope you will find that this cookbook will help you with your food selection and keep you on your prescribed diet.

Mary Jane Finsand

Sugar & Sugar Replacements

Most sweeteners or sugar replacements can be found in your supermarket. They vary in sweetness, aftertaste, aroma, and calories. The listing below is by ingredient name rather than product name. Check the side of the box or bottle to determine the contents of the product.

Aspartame and aspartame products are fairly new additions to the supermarket. Aspartame is a natural protein sweetener. Because of its intense sweetness, it reduces calories and carbohydrates in the diet. Aspartame has a sweet aroma and no aftertaste. It seems to complement some of the other sweeteners by removing their bitter aftertaste. Aspartame does lose some of its sweetness in heating and is therefore recommended for use in cold products.

Cyclamates and products containing cyclamates are not as sweet as saccharin and saccharin products, and also leave a bitter aftertaste. Many sugar replacements consist of a combination of saccharin and cyclamates.

Fructose is commonly known as fruit sugar. It is actually a natural sugar found in fruits and honey. Fructose tastes the same as common table sugar (sucrose), but because of its intense sweetness it reduces calories and carbohydrates in the diet. It is not affected by heating or cooling, but baked products made with fructose tend to be heavier.

Glycyrrhizen and products containing glycyrrhizen are as sweet as saccharin and saccharin products. They are seen less in supermarkets because they tend to give food a licorice taste and aroma.

Saccharin and products containing saccharin are the most widely known and used intense sweeteners. When used in baking or cooking, saccharin has a lingering bitter aftertaste. You will normally find it in the form of sodium saccharin in products labelled low-calorie sugar replacements. Granular, or dry, sugar replacements containing sodium saccharin give less of an aftertaste to foods that are heated. But it's best to use liquid sugar replacements containing sodium saccharin in cold foods or in foods that have partially cooled and no longer need any heating.

Sorbitol is used in many commercial food products. It has little or no aftertaste and a sweet aroma. At present it can only be bought in bulk form at health-food outlets.

Stevia Rebaudiana is a new herb sweetener that is hundreds of times sweeter than common table sugar. It comes in powdered form and is completely natural. The powder easily mixes in water to dilute its extreme sweetness. *To make liquid Stevia Rebaudiana, dissolve ¼ t. (1 mL) of the powder in ¼ c. (60 mL) of water.*

If you have difficulty finding these products, you can try contacting a distributor or mail-order outlet.

For the individual consumer, write:

The Fruitful Yield
2111 N. Bloomingdale Road
Glendale Hts, IL 60139

or

T & K Health Foods
1429 West 3rd St.
Waterloo, IA 50701

For health-food retailers or other large orders, write or call:

NOW Natural Foods
2000 Bloomingdale Road, Unit 250
Glendale Hts, IL 60139
Phone: (708) 893–1330

Using the Recipes—
Conversion Guides,
Flavorings & Extracts,
Spices & Herbs

All the recipes have been developed using granulated or liquid sugar replacements. All use a sugar replacement that has the same amount of sweetness as regular sugar. If you use a stronger product, use it in proportion to the equivalencies of that product. Remember, do not bake with an aspartame sweetener.

Read the recipes carefully; then assemble all equipment and ingredients. Use standard measuring equipment (whether metric or customary), and be sure to measure accurately.

Customary Terms

t.	teaspoon	qt.	quart
T.	tablespoon	oz.	ounce
c.	cup	lb.	pound
pkg.	package	°F	degrees Fahrenheit
pt.	pint	in.	inch

Metric Symbols

mL	millilitre	°C	degrees Celsius
L	litre	mm	millimetre
g	gram	cm	centimetre
kg	kilogram		

Guide to Approximate Equivalents

Customary				Metric	
Ounces Pounds	Cups	Tablespoons	Teaspoons	Millilitres	Grams Kilograms
			¼ t.	1 mL	1 g
			½ t.	2 mL	
			1 t.	5 mL	
			2 t.	10 mL	
½ oz.		1 T.	3 t.	15 mL	15 g
1 oz.		2 T.	6 t.	30 mL	30 g
2 oz.	¼ c.	4 T.	12 t.	60 mL	
4 oz.	½ c.	8 T.	24 t.	125 mL	
8 oz.	1 c.	16 T.	48 t.	250 mL	
2.2 lb.					1 kg

Keep in mind that this guide does not show exact conversions, but it can be used in a general way for food measurement.

Conversion Guide for Cooking Pans and Casseroles

Customary	Metric
1 qt.	1 L
2 qt.	2 L
3 qt.	3 L

Candy-Thermometer Guide

Use this guide to test for doneness.

Fahrenheit °F	Test		Celsius °C
230–234°	Syrup:	Thread	100–112°
234–240°	Fondant/Fudge:	Soft ball	112–115°
244–248°	Caramels:	Firm ball	118–120°
250–266°	Marshmallows:	Hard Ball	121–130°
270–290°	Taffy:	Soft crack	132–143°
300–310°	Brittle:	Hard crack	149–154°

Oven-Cooking Guides

Fahrenheit °F	Oven Heat	Celsius °C
250–275°	very slow	120–135°
300–325°	slow	150–165°
350–375°	moderate	175–190°
400–425°	hot	200–220°
450–475°	very hot	230–245°
475–500°	hottest	250–290°

Guide to Baking-Pan Sizes

Customary	Metric	Holds	Holds (Metric)
8-in. pie	20-cm pie	2 c.	600 mL
9-in. pie	23-cm pie	1 qt.	1 L
10-in. pie	25-cm pie	1¼ qt.	1.3 L
8-in. round	20-cm round	1 qt.	1 L
9-in. round	23-cm round	1½ qt.	1.5 L
8-in. square	20-cm square	2 qt.	2 L
9-in. square	23-cm square	2½ qt.	2.5 L
9 × 5 × 2 in. loaf	23 × 13 × 5 cm loaf	2 qt.	2 L
9-in. tube	23-cm tube	3 qt.	3 L
10-in. tube	25-cm tube	3 qt.	3 L
10-in. Bundt	25-cm Bundt	3 qt.	3 L
9 × 5 in.	23 × 13 cm	1½ qt.	1.5 L
10 × 6 in.	25 × 16 cm	3½ qt.	3.5 L
11 × 7 in.	27 × 17 cm	3½ qt.	3.5 L
13 × 9 × 2 in.	33 × 23 × 5 cm	3½ qt.	3.5 L
14 × 10 in.	36 × 25 cm	cookie tin	
15½ × 10½ × 1 in.	39 × 25 × 3 cm	jelly roll	

Flavorings and Extracts

Orange, lime, and lemon peels give pastries and puddings a fresh, clean flavor. Liquor flavors, such as brandy and rum, give cakes and other desserts a company flair. Choose from the following to give your recipes some zip, without adding calories.

Almond	Butter rum	Pecan
Anise (Licorice)	Cherry	Peppermint
Apricot	Chocolate	Pineapple
Banana creme	Coconut	Raspberry
Blackberry	Grape	Rum
Black walnut	Hazelnut	Sassafras
Blueberry	Lemon	Sherry
Brandy	Lime	Strawberry
Butter	Mint	Vanilla
Butternut	Orange	Walnut

Spices and Herbs

These are some of my favorite spices and herbs. They will definitely add distinction to your desserts, without adding calories.

Allspice: cinnamon, ginger, and nutmeg flavor; used in breads, pastries, jellies, jams, and pickles.

Anise: licorice flavor; used in candies, breads, fruit, wine, and liqueurs.

Cinnamon: pungent, sweet flavor; used in pastries, breads, pickles, wine, beer, and liqueurs.

Clove: pungent, sweet flavor; used in ham, sauces, pastries, puddings, fruit, wine, and liqueurs.

Coriander: bitter-lemon flavor; used in cookies, cakes, pies, puddings, fruit, and wine and liqueur punches.

Ginger: strong, pungent flavor; used in anything sweet, also with beer, brandy, and liqueurs.

Nutmeg: sweet, nutty flavor; used in pastries, puddings, and vegetables.

Woodruff: sweet, vanilla flavor; used in wines and punches.

Tips & Tricks from My Kitchen

I cannot express enough the importance of using heavy bakeware. Heavy bakeware absorbs, retains, and distributes heat evenly. Many of the lighter-weight cake pans and cookie sheets have dead or hot spots in them. I find that in cooking with fructose, a heavy, very shiny aluminum surface produces the best, most uniform desserts.

While I do use the newer dark bakeware, I rarely consider that any bakeware with a synthetic self-releasing or nonstick surface truly has a nonstick surface. Also, I find that the dark bakeware requires different baking temperatures and times. (Remember, dark colors absorb heat.) So, if you do use dark bakeware, you might want to lower the temperature and watch your item very closely near the end of its baking time. Because I have a tendency to scratch the bottom and sides of pans, nonstick pans don't last as long for me. In addition, I find that products baked in the darker bakeware are smaller, heavier, and crispier than I want.

It is important that baking sheets or pans be kept clean and free from burns. Burned surfaces on baking sheets or pans prevent heat from distributing evenly, causing baked products to brown improperly. Items baked on burned sheets can come out of the oven underdone, overdone, or burned.

When baking a cake, use a heavy aluminum pan. Line the bottom with wax paper, and don't grease or flour the sides. Fill the pan and bake as directed. After allowing the cake to cool slightly, release the sides by running a flexible spatula between the edges of the pan and the cake. Try to keep the edge of the spatula pressed tightly against the sides of the pan. Place a rack over the pan and invert. Remove the wax paper, place another rack over the cake, and invert. Allow the cake to cool completely.

The easiest way of cutting a cake into layers is to mark the layer by sticking toothpicks around the cake at the level you want the layer. Then use a long, sharp knife or a piece of thread to cut through the cake at that level. If you are making three layers, mark and cut each layer separately.

Many cookware sets don't come with a double boiler. A double boiler consists of two pans, with the top pan sitting on the bottom pan. A simple double boiler can be made by placing a heat-proof bowl over a saucepan. The water in the bottom of the double boiler should not boil, just simmer.

I find that when I cook instant puddings, a wire whisk produces the best results.

If you don't have a food processor or blender and want to chop an ingredient such as nuts, use a heavy knife. If you want to crush crackers or dry bread into crumbs, place broken pieces into a plastic bag and crush with your hand or a rolling pin.

You don't need a crepe iron to make crepes; a 6-in. frying pan will work. Heat a pan lightly sprayed with vegetable oil. Then remove the pan and place about 1 T. (15 mL) of batter in the pan, curl the pan until the batter coats the bottom, return to the heat, and fry lightly.

Drinks

Chocolate Mint Dessert Drink

2 c.	low-fat ice cream	500 mL
2 T.	chocolate flavoring or extract	30 mL
2 T.	mint flavoring or extract	30 mL
1 T.	chunky peanut butter	15 mL
4	fresh mint sprigs (optional)	4

Combine the ice cream, flavorings, and peanut butter in a blender. Blend until smooth and creamy. Pour into four wine glasses. If desired, garnish each with a mint sprig.

Yield: 4 servings
Exchange, 1 serving: 1 low-fat milk
Calories, 1 serving: 116
Carbohydrates, 1 serving: 15 g

Tropical Punch

1 c.	mango nectar	250 mL
1 c.	unsweetened pineapple juice	250 mL
¾ c.	guava nectar	190 mL
¼ c.	lime juice	60 mL
6½ c.	cracked ice	1625 mL

Mix juices in a large pitcher. Combine 1 c. (250 mL) of the punch with 2 c. (500 mL) of the cracked ice in a blender. Blend until smooth. Pour into two glasses. Repeat procedure with remaining punch in batches.

Yield: 6 servings
Exchange, 1 serving: 1 fruit
Calories, 1 serving: 69
Carbohydrates, 1 serving: 17 g

Party Pineapple Punch

2	bananas	2
3 c.	unsweetened pineapple juice	750 mL
6-oz. can	orange-juice concentrate	178-g can
3 c.	cold water	750 mL
2 T.	lemon juice	30 mL
5 env.	aspartame sweetener	5 env.
1 bottle	diet lemon-lime soda	1 bottle
(1-qt.)		(1-L)

Cut bananas into chunks and place in a blender. Add 1 c. (250 mL) of the pineapple juice and orange-juice concentrate. Blend until smooth. Transfer to large bowl. Add the remaining 2 c. (500 mL) of the pineapple juice and the cold water, lemon juice, and aspartame sweetener. Stir to completely mix. Pour into a large metal baking pan. Place in freezer and allow to freeze into a slush. Scoop into a punch bowl. Pour the lemon-lime soda down the sides of the bowl. Stir gently to mix. Serve in small punch cups.

Yield: 24 servings
Exchange, 1 serving: ⅔ fruit
Calories, 1 serving: 39
Carbohydrates, 1 serving: 9 g

Double-Raspberry Cooler

1½ c.	cracked ice	375 mL
1½ c.	fresh or frozen unsweetened raspberries	190 mL
4	thin slices of lemon	4
6 T.	low-calorie raspberry syrup	90 mL
2 c.	sparkling water	500 mL

Divide cracked ice and raspberries equally among four glasses. Add one lemon slice, 1½ T. (21 mL) of raspberry syrup, and ½ c. (125 mL) of sparkling water to each glass. Serve with spoons so that the fruit can be muddled.

Yield: 4 servings
Exchange, 1 serving: ¾ fruit
Calories, 1 serving: 43
Carbohydrates, 1 serving: 10 g

Mango Cooler

1 lb.	mango	500 g
½ c.	fresh lemon juice	125 mL
1 T.	rum flavoring	15 mL
1 T.	granulated fructose	15 mL
	or	
6 env.	aspartame sweetener	6 env.
3 c.	cracked ice	750 mL

Peel, pit, and chop mango. Place mango pieces in a blender and process to a puree. Add lemon juice, rum flavoring, and sweetener of your choice. Then add the cracked ice and blend until smooth. Pour into chilled glasses.

Yield: 4 servings
Exchange, 1 serving: 1 fruit
Calories, 1 serving: 50
Carbohydrates, 1 serving: 12

Cranberry Grapefruit Cooler

3 c.	unsweetened pink-grapefruit juice	3 c.
2½ c.	low-calorie cranberry-juice cocktail	625 mL
2 T.	granulated sugar replacement	30 mL
	or	
5 env.	aspartame sweetener	5 env.
3 c.	cracked ice	750 mL
6	thin slices of lime	6

Combine pink-grapefruit juice, cranberry juice, and sweetener of your choice in a large pitcher. Stir to dissolve sweetener. Divide the cracked ice equally among six glasses. Pour juice mixture into glasses. Garnish each glass with a slice of lime. This makes a perfect dessert drink after a barbecue dinner on a warm night.

Yield: 6 servings
Exchange, 1 serving: 1 fruit
Calories, 1 serving: 63
Carbohydrates, 1 serving: 16 g

Strawberry Slush

1½ c.	frozen, unsweetened whole strawberries	375 mL
½ c.	buttermilk	125 mL
1 T.	granulated fructose	15 mL

Allow strawberries to thaw slightly. Reserve one or two of the larger strawberries. Combine buttermilk and fructose in a blender or food processor. With the motor running, gradually add the strawberries (keeping top of blender covered to prevent splashing). Process into a slush. Pour into a decorative glass. Cut reserved strawberries into medium-sized pieces. Stir into strawberry slush.

Yield: 1 serving
Exchange: 1 fruit, ½ skim milk
Calories: 105
Carbohydrates: 21 g

Orange Sipper

1½ c.	buttermilk	375 mL
⅓ c.	orange-juice concentrate, undiluted	90 mL
¾ t.	liquid Stevia Rebaudiana extract (page 8)	7 mL
	or	
2 T.	granulated sugar replacement	30 mL
1 t.	vanilla extract	5 mL
3	ice cubes	3

Combine buttermilk, orange-juice concentrate, sweetener of your choice, and vanilla. Blend until completely mixed. With blender running, drop ice cubes, one at a time, into the liquid. Blend until smooth. (Extra amount of drink can be frozen for later use. Place in freezer container. Allow to thaw slightly before using, then process in blender.)

Yield: 4 servings
Exchange, 1 serving: ⅔ skim milk, ½ fruit
Calories, 1 serving: 87
Carbohydrates, 1 serving: 17 g

Peach Slush

1½ c.	frozen, unsweetened peach slices	375 mL
½ c.	skim milk	125 mL
3 env.	aspartame sweetener	3 env.
1	fresh mint sprig (optional)	1

Allow peach slices to thaw slightly. Pour milk into a blender or food processor. With the motor running, gradually add the peach slices (keeping top of blender covered to prevent splashing). Process into a slush. Blend in aspartame sweetener. Pour into a decorative glass. If desired, garnish with a sprig of mint.

Yield: 1 serving
Exchange: 1½ fruit, ½ skim milk
Calories: 143
Carbohydrates: 30 g

Peach Smoothie

1¼ c.	nonfat plain yogurt	310 mL
1 lb.	ripe peaches	500 g
2 T.	fresh lemon juice	30 mL
2 T.	liquid fructose	30 mL
¼ t.	vanilla extract	1 mL

Divide 1 c. (250 mL) of the yogurt among 8 to 10 sections of an ice-cube tray. Freeze hard (at least 4 to 5 hours). Peel, pit, and slice peaches. Combine peach slices and lemon juice in a blender. Process until almost a puree. Add the remaining ¼ c. yogurt and the liquid fructose and vanilla. Process into a puree. Add frozen yogurt cubes and process until smooth. Pour into four decorative glasses.

Yield: 4 servings
Exchange, 1 serving: 1 fruit, ½ skim milk
Calories, 1 serving: 81
Carbohydrates, 1 serving: 16 g

Strawberry Yogurt Nog

1½ c.	fresh or frozen unsweetened strawberries	375 mL
1½ c.	skim milk	375 mL
8 oz.	nonfat plain yogurt	227 g
1 t.	vanilla extract	5 mL
1 t.	strawberry flavoring	5 mL
6 env.	aspartame sweetener	6 env.
	or	
1 T.	granulated fructose	15 mL
3	ice cubes	3

(If you are using fresh strawberries, you might want to set four aside for garnish.) Combine strawberries, milk, yogurt, vanilla extract, strawberry flavoring, and sweetener of your choice in a blender. Process until smooth. With the motor running, add ice cubes, one at a time, through the feed tube in the lid. Blend until smooth. Pour into decorative red-wine glasses. (Cut reserved fresh strawberries into a fan. Lay on top of nog.)

Yield: 4 servings
Exchange, 1 serving: 1 skim milk
Calories, 1 serving: 76
Carbohydrates, 1 serving: 10 g

Black-Raspberry Tofu Cream

1 c.	fresh or frozen black raspberries	250 mL
½ c.	skim milk	125 mL
1 t.	vanilla extract	5 mL
3 env.	aspartame sweetener	3 env.
½ pkg.	firm tofu	½ pkg.
(10.5-oz.)		(297-g)

Combine black raspberries and skim milk in a blender. Process until smooth. Add vanilla and aspartame sweetener. Process to mix. Add tofu. Process until smooth. Pour into two white-wine glasses.

Yield: 2 servings
Exchange, 1 serving: 1 skim milk, 1 medium-fat meat
Calories, 1 serving: 157
Carbohydrates, 1 serving: 14 g

Banana Yogurt Nog

1	banana	1
1½ c.	skim milk	375 mL
8 oz.	nonfat plain yogurt	227 g
2 t.	vanilla extract	10 mL
4 env.	aspartame sweetener	4 env.
	or	
1½ T.	granulated sugar replacement	21 mL
3	ice cubes	3

Combine banana, milk, yogurt, vanilla extract, and sweetener of your choice in a blender. Process until smooth. With the motor running, add ice cubes, one at a time, through the feed tube in the lid. Blend until smooth. Pour into decorative red-wine glasses.

Yield: 4 servings
Exchange, 1 serving: 1 skim milk
Calories, 1 serving: 86
Carbohydrates, 1 serving: 14 g

Banana Tofu Cream

½ c.	skim milk	125 mL
1	banana	1
1 t.	vanilla extract	5 mL
3 env.	aspartame sweetener	3 env.
½ pkg.	firm tofu	½ pkg.
(10.5-oz.)		(297-g)
	ground nutmeg	

Combine skim milk and banana in a blender. Process until smooth. Add vanilla and aspartame sweetener. Process to mix. Add tofu. Process until smooth. Pour into two white-wine glasses. (A champagne flute can also be used.) Sprinkle surface with nutmeg.

Yield: 2 servings
Exchange, 1 serving: 1½ skim milk, 1 fat
Calories, 1 serving: 122
Carbohydrates, 1 serving: 18 g

Hot Cider

2 c.	apple cider	500 mL
2	cinnamon sticks	2
(3-in.)		(7.5-cm)
½ t.	whole cloves	2 mL
⅛ t.	ground nutmeg	½ mL
2 env.	aspartame sweetener	2 env.
2 t.	rum flavoring	10 mL

In a small saucepan, heat the apple cider, cinnamon sticks, whole cloves, and nutmeg until boiling. Reduce heat and simmer gently for 5 to 6 minutes. Remove from heat; then remove cinnamon sticks and whole cloves. Stir in aspartame sweetener and rum flavoring. Pour into two preheated cups or mugs. (To preheat mugs: Pour boiling or very hot water into mugs, allow to stand for 1 to 2 minutes, then pour out hot water and fill with drink.)

Yield: 2 servings
Exchange, 1 serving: 1 fruit
Calories, 1 serving: 100
Carbohydrates, 1 serving: 13 g

Coffee and Cream

1 env.	nondairy whipped-topping powder	1 env.
(2 c.)		(2 c.)
3 T.	lemon juice	45 mL
2 T.	water	30 mL
4 env.	aspartame sweetener	4 env.
1 T.	instant-coffee powder	15 mL
2 c.	cracked ice	500 mL
1 c.	diet ginger ale	250 mL

Combine whipped-topping powder, lemon juice, water, aspartame sweetener, and instant-coffee powder in a blender. Process until foamy. Add ice and process using the off/on switch until smooth. Add ginger ale and process on LOW until blended.

Yield: 6 servings
Exchange, 1 serving: 1 fat, ¼ fruit
Calories, 1 serving: 62
Carbohydrates, 1 serving: 6 g

Quick Cappuccino

3 c.	hot strong coffee*	750 mL
3 c.	scalded skim milk	750 mL
12 env.	aspartame sweetener	12 env.
	unsweetened cocoa powder	

*To brew strong coffee, use double the amount of coffee that you would normally use.

Pour scalded milk into a blender. Place hot pad over blender cover to protect yourself against burning. Process the milk until frothy. Pour ½ c. (500 mL) of the strong coffee into each of six cups or mugs. Pour ½ c. (500 mL) of the hot milk into each of the cups. Stir two envelopes of aspartame sweetener into each cup. Sprinkle with a small amount of unsweetened cocoa. Serve immediately.

Yield: 6 servings
Exchange, 1 serving: ½ low-fat milk
Calories, 1 serving: 50
Carbohydrates, 1 serving: 6 g

Prince Alex After-Dinner Drink

2 T.	water	30 mL
2 T.	low-fat ice cream	30 mL
1 T.	liquid nondairy creamer	15 mL
1 t.	chocolate flavoring	5 mL
	ground nutmeg	

Shake ingredients (except nutmeg) with ice cubes in a shaker jar. Place one ice cube into a chilled cocktail glass. Strain mixture over ice cube in glass. Dust with nutmeg.

Yield: 1 serving
Exchange: negligible
Calories: negligible
Carbohydrates: negligible

Ices & Sherbets

Pineapple Sherbet

3¼ c.	unsweetened pineapple juice	875 mL
¼ c.	crushed pineapple in juice	60 mL
1 env.	unflavored gelatin	1 env.
⅛ t.	Stevia Rebaudiana extract	½ mL
	or	
5 env.	aspartame sweetener	5 env.
1 c.	low-fat milk	250 mL

In a saucepan, mix pineapple juice, crushed pineapple with juice, unflavored gelatin, and Stevia Rebaudiana extract. Cook and stir until gelatin and Stevia Rebaudiana are dissolved and mixture is slightly warmed. Remove from heat. Stir in milk. (Mixture will appear to have curdled slightly.) Mix all ingredients. Freeze in an ice-cream freezer, according to manufacturer's directions, or pour mixture into a 9-in. (23-cm) baking pan and place pan in freezer for 2 to 3 hours or until mixture is almost firm. Remove pan from freezer and break pineapple mixture into pieces. Place pieces in a chilled bowl. Beat with an electric mixer until smooth but not melted. Transfer back to pan. Cover and freeze until firm.

Yield: 8 servings
Exchange, 1 serving: 1 fruit
Calories, 1 serving: 76
Carbohydrates, 1 serving: 15 g

Grape Sherbet

½ c.	grape juice	125 mL
½ c.	low-fat milk	125 mL

| ½ t. | vanilla extract | 2 mL |
| ⅓ c. | prepared nondairy whipped topping | 90 mL |

Combine grape juice, milk, and vanilla in a bowl. (Mixture will appear to have curdled slightly.) Stir to combine ingredients. Place bowl in freezer and chill until mixture is almost firm. Remove bowl from freezer and break mixture into pieces. Beat with an electric mixer until smooth but not melted. Beat in nondairy whipped topping. Cover and freeze to desired consistency.

Yield: 2 servings
Exchange, 1 serving: ½ fruit, ½ low-fat milk
Calories, 1 serving: 108
Carbohydrates, 1 serving: 13 g

Strawberry Sorbet

1 env.	unflavored gelatin	1 env.
1½ c.	cool water	375 mL
1-lb. pkg.	frozen strawberries, slightly thawed	454-g pkg.
½ c.	reduced-calorie cranberry-juice cocktail	125 mL
1 T.	liquid Stevia Rebaudiana extract (page 8)	15 mL
	or	
½ c.	granulated sugar replacement	125 mL
2 T.	lemon juice	30 mL

In a medium-sized saucepan, sprinkle gelatin over cool water. Allow to soften for 1 minute. Cook and stir over low heat until gelatin has dissolved. Cool to room temperature. Meanwhile, combine strawberries and cranberry-juice cocktail in a blender or food processor. Process to a puree. Blend in sweetener of your choice and lemon juice. When gelatin has cooled, blend into strawberry mixture. Pour into a 9-in (23-cm) baking pan; freeze until firm (about 3 hours). Break into pieces. Place in a large mixing bowl or food processor. With an electric mixer or food processor, beat mixture until smooth. Return to pan and refreeze. Before serving, allow sorbet to stand at room temperature for about 15 minutes or until slightly softened.

Yield: 8 servings
Exchange, 1 serving: ⅓ fruit
Calories, 1 serving: 24
Carbohydrates, 1 serving: 4 g

Orange Sherbet

3½ c.	orange juice	875 mL
1 env.	unflavored gelatin	1 env.
⅛ t.	Stevia Rebaudiana extract	½ mL
	or	
5 env.	aspartame sweetener	5 env.
1 c.	low-fat milk	250 mL
	orange food coloring*	

*If you don't have orange food coloring, combine red and yellow to make orange.

In a saucepan, mix orange juice, unflavored gelatin, and Stevia Rebaudiana extract. Cook and stir until gelatin and Stevia Rebaudiana are dissolved and mixture is slightly warmed. Remove from heat. Stir in milk. (Mixture will appear to have curdled slightly.) Mix all ingredients. Freeze in an ice-cream freezer, according to manufacturer's directions, or pour mixture into a 9-in. (23-cm) baking pan and place pan in freezer for 2 to 3 hours or until mixture is almost firm. Remove pan from freezer and break mixture into pieces. Place pieces in a chilled bowl. Beat with an electric mixer until smooth but not melted. Transfer back to pan. Cover and freeze until firm.

Yield: 8 servings
Exchange, 1 serving: 1 fruit
Calories, 1 serving: 62
Carbohydrates, 1 serving: 14 g

Blackberry Buttermilk Sherbet

1-lb. bag	frozen, unsweetened blackberries	454-g bag
1	egg	1
dash	salt	dash
⅛ t.	Stevia Rebaudiana extract	½ mL
	or	
5 env.	aspartame sweetener	5 env.
2 c.	buttermilk	500 mL

Slightly thaw blackberries. Transfer to a food processor or blender and process to puree. Set aside. Separate egg, setting the white aside. Combine egg yolk, salt, and Stevia Rebaudiana extract in a bowl. Beat until thick and lemon-colored. Gradually beat in blackberry puree. Blend in buttermilk. Beat egg white until it holds a firm peak. Fold buttermilk-blackberry mixture into beaten egg white just enough to blend. Transfer mixture to an ice-cream freezer and freeze according to manufacturer's directions, or pour mixture into a 9-in. (23-cm) baking pan and place pan in freezer for 2 to 3 hours or until mixture is almost firm. Remove pan from freezer and break mixture into pieces. Place pieces in a chilled bowl. Beat with an electric mixer until smooth but not melted. Transfer back to pan. Cover and freeze until firm.

Yield: 10 servings
Exchange, 1 serving: 1 fruit
Calories, 1 serving: 52
Carbohydrates, 1 serving: 13 g

Lemon Sherbet

3 c.	water	750 mL
1 env.	unflavored gelatin	1 env.
⅛ t.	Stevia Rebaudiana extract	½ mL
	or	
5 env.	aspartame sweetener	5 env.
¾ c.	fresh lemon juice	190 mL
1 c.	low-fat milk	250 mL
1 t.	grated lemon peel	5 mL

In a saucepan, mix water, unflavored gelatin, and Stevia Rebaudiana extract. Cook and stir until gelatin and Stevia Rebaudiana are dissolved and mixture is slightly warmed. Remove from heat. Stir in lemon juice, milk, and lemon peel. (Mixture will appear to have curdled slightly.) Mix all ingredients. Freeze in an ice-cream freezer, according to manufacturer's directions, or pour mixture into a 9-in. (23-cm) baking pan and place pan in freezer for 2 to 3 hours or until mixture is almost firm. Remove pan from freezer and break mixture into pieces. Place pieces in a chilled bowl, and beat with an electric mixer until smooth but not melted. Or process pieces in a food processor in small batches using the pulse or on/off switch. Transfer back to pan. Cover and freeze until firm.

Yield: 8 servings
Exchange, 1 serving: negligible
Calories, 1 serving: 15
Carbohydrates, 1 serving: negligible

Quick Orange-Yogurt Pops

6-oz. can	orange-juice concentrate	210-g can
¾ c.	water	190 mL
1 c.	plain low-fat yogurt	250 mL

Combine ingredients in a blender. Process until well blended. Divide mixture evenly among eight paper drinking cups. Place in freezer and freeze until frozen. If desired, when pops are partially frozen, place a wooden stick in middle of each pop. Freeze completely.

Yield: 8 servings
Exchange, 1 serving: 1 fruit
Calories, 1 serving: 68
Carbohydrates, 1 serving: 9 g

Blueberry Tofu Cream

1½ c.	fresh or unsweetened frozen blueberries	375 mL
2 t.	lemon juice	10 mL
1 env.	unflavored gelatin	1 env.
⅓ c.	water	90 mL
⅔ c.	granulated sugar replacement	180 mL
	or	
⅓ c.	granulated fructose	90 mL
	or	
1 T.	liquid Stevia Rebaudiana extract (page 8)	15 mL
½ pkg.	tofu, firm	½ pkg.
(10.5-oz.)		(297-g)
1½ c.	low-fat milk	375 mL
1 T.	vanilla extract	15 mL
½ c.	prepared nondairy whipped topping	125 mL

Puree blueberries in a blender. Transfer to a heavy saucepan, and bring to a boil. Reduce heat and simmer, uncovered, until blueberries are reduced to about ½ c. (125 mL). Stir in lemon juice and cool to room temperature. In a small saucepan, sprinkle gelatin over water. Allow to soften for 1 minute. Cook and stir over low heat until gelatin dissolves. Set aside to cool. When the gelatin is cooled, combine gelatin, water, sweetener of your choice, and tofu in a blender. Blend until smooth. Pour in milk and vanilla. Blend until completely mixed. Add nondairy whipped topping and pureed blueberries. Blend just until mixed. Transfer to an ice-cream freezer or a 9-in. (23-cm) baking pan. Freeze according to freezer manufacturer's instructions or place pan in the freezer and freeze until firm. Break into pieces. Place in a large mixing bowl or food processor. With an electric mixer or food processor, beat mixture until smooth. Return to the pan and refreeze. To serve: Score into eight equal servings, and place on chilled serving plates. Serve immediately (Tofu Cream softens quickly).

Yield: 8 servings, with granulated sugar replacement or liquid Stevia Rebaudiana
Exchange, 1 serving: ½ fruit, ⅓ low-fat milk
Calories, 1 serving: 50
Carbohydrates, 1 serving: 7 g

Yield: 8 servings, with granulated fructose
Exchange, 1 serving: ⅔ fruit, ½ low-fat milk
Calories, 1 serving: 92
Carbohydrates, 1 serving: 17 g

Watermelon Sorbet

1 env.	unflavored gelatin	1 env.
1½ c.	cool water	375 mL
1½ qt.	watermelon cut in 1-in. (2.5-cm) chunks	1½ L
1 T	liquid Stevia Rebaudiana extract (page 8)	15 mL
	or	
½ c.	granulated sugar replacement	125 mL
2 T.	lemon juice	30 mL.

In a medium-sized saucepan, sprinkle gelatin over cool water. Allow to soften for 1 minute. Cook and stir over low heat until gelatin has dissolved. Cool to room temperature. Meanwhile, puree watermelon chunks in a blender or food processor. Blend in sweetener of your choice and lemon juice. When gelatin has cooled, blend into watermelon mixture. Pour into a 9-in. (23-cm) baking pan; freeze until firm (about 3 hours). Break into pieces. Place in a large mixing bowl or food processor. With an electric mixer or food processor, beat mixture until smooth. Return to pan and refreeze. Before serving, allow sorbet to stand at room temperature for about 15 minutes or until slightly softened.

Yield: 8 servings
Exchange, 1 serving: ½ fruit
Calories, 1 serving: 30
Carbohydrates, 1 serving: 7 g

Cranberry Ice

1 lb.	fresh cranberries	500 g
1½ c.	water	375 mL
¾ c.	granulated sugar replacement	190 mL
	or	
½ c.	granulated fructose	125 mL
	or	
⅛ t.	Stevia Rebaudiana extract	½ mL
⅓ c.	orange juice	90 mL
1 T.	lemon juice	15 mL

Combine cranberries and water in a saucepan. Cook uncovered until berries have "popped." Remove from heat and stir in sweetener of your choice, orange juice, and lemon juice. Transfer to a blender or food processor. Process until smooth. If still warm, cool to room temperature. Pour mixture into a 9-in. (23-cm) baking pan. Freeze until firm. Remove from freezer and allow to stand at room temperature for 5 to 6 minutes. Break cranberry mixture into pieces and transfer to a large mixing bowl or food processor. Whip or process until smooth. Serve immediately or cover and refreeze. Before serving, allow mixture to stand at room temperature until slightly softened. Then scoop into eight decorative glasses or bowls. (This dessert can also be frozen, in either eight paper drinking cups or eight cup-cake cups lined with plastic wrap. At serving time, remove from cups.)

Yield: 8 servings, with granulated sugar replacement or Stevia
Rebaudiana
Exchange, 1 serving: negligible
Calories, 1 serving: negligible
Carbohydrates, 1 serving: negligible

Yield: 8 servings, with granulated fructose
Exchange, 1 serving: 1 fruit
Calories, 1 serving: 48
Carbohydrates, 1 serving: 13 g

Strawberry Ice

1 qt.	fresh or frozen unsweetened strawberries	1 L
½ c.	water	125 mL
½ c.	granulated sugar replacement	125 mL
	or	
¼ c.	granulated fructose	60 mL

	or	
1 T.	liquid Stevia Rebaudiana extract (page 8)	15 mL
2 T.	lemon juice	30 mL

In a food processor or blender, process strawberries into a puree. Add water, sweetener of your choice, and lemon juice. Process to mix. Pour mixture into a 9-in. (23-cm) baking pan. Freeze until firm. Remove from freezer and allow to stand at room temperature for 5 to 6 minutes. Break strawberry mixture into pieces and transfer to a large mixing bowl or food processor. Whip or process until smooth. Serve immediately or cover and refreeze. Before serving, allow mixture to stand at room temperature until slightly softened. Then scoop into six decorative glasses or bowls. (This dessert can also be frozen, in either six paper drinking cups or six cupcake cups lined with plastic wrap. At serving time, remove from cups.)

Yield: 6 servings, with granulated sugar replacement or liquid Stevia
  Rebaudiana
Exchange, 1 serving: ⅔ fruit
Calories, 1 serving: 36
Carbohydrates, 1 serving: 8 g

Yield: 6 servings, with granulated fructose
Exchange, 1 serving: 1 fruit
Calories, 1 serving: 52
Carbohydrates, 1 serving: 12 g

Tart-Cherry Ice Cream

| 2 qts. | vanilla ice cream | 2 L |
| 1-lb. bag | frozen, unsweetened, pitted tart red cherries | 456-g bag |

Soften the ice cream in the refrigerator until it can be whipped with an electric beater. Meanwhile, thaw, drain, and pat the cherries dry with paper towels. Transfer the ice cream to a large mixing bowl. Whip the ice cream on LOW until smooth. Fold in the cherries. Transfer the ice cream to a covered freezer container. Freeze for several hours before serving. If the ice cream becomes solid, soften it slightly in the refrigerator before serving.

Yield: 16 servings
Exchange, 1 serving: 1 bread
Calories, 1 serving: 98
Carbohydrates, 1 serving: 15 g

Fresh Raspberry Ice Cream

2 qts.	vanilla ice cream	2 L
1 qt.	fresh raspberries	1 L
1 T.	granulated fructose	15 mL

Soften the ice cream in the refrigerator until it can be whipped with an electric beater. Wash and clean the raspberries. Transfer to a medium-sized bowl. With a fork, slightly crush raspberries. Sprinkle with fructose. Stir, cover, and allow to rest 30 minutes. Transfer the ice cream to a large mixing bowl. Whip the ice cream on LOW until smooth. Fold in the crushed raspberries, allowing the raspberries to marbleize the ice cream. Transfer the ice cream to a covered freezer container. Freeze for several hours before serving. If the ice cream becomes solid, soften it slightly in the refrigerator before serving.

Yield: 16 servings
Exchange, 1 serving: 1 bread, ½ fruit
Calories, 1 serving: 121
Carbohydrates, 1 serving: 21 g

Fresh Apple Cinnamon Ice Cream

2 T.	margarine	30 mL
3 large	Red Delicious apples	3 large
	(peeled, cored, and chopped)	
2 in.	cinnamon stick	5 cm
2 qts.	vanilla ice cream	2 L

Melt margarine in a heavy skillet over medium heat. Add apples and cinnamon stick. Sauté for 5 minutes. Remove from heat and cool completely. Soften the ice cream in the refrigerator until it can be whipped with an electric beater. Transfer the ice cream to a large mixing bowl. Whip the ice cream on LOW until smooth. Remove cinnamon stick. Fold the apple mixture into the ice cream. Transfer to a covered freezer container. Freeze for several hours before serving. If the ice cream becomes solid, soften it slightly in the refrigerator before serving.

Yield: 16 servings
Exchange, 1 serving: 1 bread, ¼ fruit
Calories, 1 serving: 110
Carbohydrates, 1 serving: 19 g

Grand Marnier Ice Cream

2 qts.	vanilla ice cream	2 L
⅓ c.	Grand Marnier	90 mL
1 recipe	candied orange peel (page 121)*	1 recipe

*The actual name of the recipe is Sweetened Citrus Peel.

Soften the ice cream in the refrigerator until it can be whipped with an electric beater. Transfer the ice cream to a large mixing bowl. Whip the ice cream on LOW until smooth. Beat in the Grand Marnier. Transfer the ice cream to a covered freezer container. Freeze for several hours before serving. If the ice cream becomes solid, soften it slightly in the refrigerator before serving. Garnish with Candied Orange Peel.

Yield: 16 servings
Exchange, 1 serving: 1½ bread
Calories, 1 serving: 135
Carbohydrates, 1 serving: 22 g

Toasted-Walnut Chocolate-Chip Ice Cream

2 qts.	vanilla ice cream	2 L
1 c.	English walnut pieces	250 mL
½ c.	mini–semisweet chocolate chips	125 mL

Soften the ice cream in the refrigerator until it can be whipped with an electric beater. Meanwhile, place walnuts in a nonstick skillet. Place over medium-low heat, and shake pan occasionally to toast the walnuts. Remove from heat and allow to cool completely. Transfer the ice cream to a large mixing bowl. Whip the ice cream on LOW until smooth. Fold in the toasted walnuts and chocolate chips. Transfer the ice cream to a covered freezer container. Freeze for several hours before serving. If the ice cream becomes solid, soften it slightly in the refrigerator before serving.

Yield: 16 servings
Exchange, 1 serving: 1 bread, 1½ fat
Calories, 1 serving: 166
Carbohydrates, 1 serving: 14 g

Frozen Desserts

Maple Ice-Cream Tart

1 qt.	reduced-calorie vanilla ice cream	1 L
½ c.	chopped toasted pecans	125 mL
2 t.	caramel flavoring	10 mL
¾ c.	sugar-free maple syrup	190 mL

Soften the ice cream just enough to stir. Stir in toasted pecans and caramel flavoring. Pack into a 9-in. (23-cm) removable-bottomed tart pan, lined with plastic wrap. Refreeze until firm. To serve: Carefully remove ice-cream tart from pan by turning it upside down on a decorative plate. Remove plastic wrap. Pour maple syrup over top of ice-cream tart. Serve immediately.

Yield: 12 servings
Exchange, 1 serving: ⅔ bread, ⅔ fat
Calories, 1 serving: 92
Carbohydrates, 1 serving: 10 g

Blueberry Mountain Dessert

1-lb. pkg.	frozen, unsweetened blueberries	456-g pkg.
5 env.	aspartame sweetener	5 env.
½ t.	lemon juice	2 mL
2⅔ c.	reduced-calorie vanilla ice cream	680 mL
8 T.	prepared nondairy whipped topping	120 mL

Remove ½ c. (125 mL) of the blueberries from the package. Set aside. Puree remaining blueberries, aspartame sweetener, and lemon juice in a food processor or blender. Pour the pureed blueberries into a heavy saucepan. Cook and stir over medium heat until mixture is very thick. Transfer to a bowl and chill for at least 30 minutes. Meanwhile, soften the ice cream. Line eight muffin or custard cups with plastic wrap. Pack each cup with ⅓ c. (90 mL) of ice cream. Freeze until firm. To serve: Turn cup upside down on a decorative plate. Remove cup and plastic wrap. Top with one-eighth of the blueberry puree. Top that with 1 T. (15 ml) of the nondairy whipped topping. Garnish with a few of the reserved blueberries. Repeat this procedure with each ice-cream cup.

Yield: 8 servings
Exchange, 1 serving: ⅔ bread, ⅔ fruit
Calories, 1 serving: 90
Carbohydrates, 1 serving: 21 g

Blackberry Lemon Parfait

1-lb. pkg.	frozen, unsweetened blackberries	456-g pkg.
5 env.	aspartame sweetener	5 env.
½ t.	lemon juice	2 mL
1 recipe	Lemon Sherbet (page 27)	1 recipe
	or	
1 qt.	reduced-calorie lemon sherbet	1 L

Puree blackberries, aspartame sweetener, and lemon juice in a food processor or blender. Measure 1¼ c. (310 ml) of the blackberry puree and place in a heavy saucepan. Reserve remaining blackberry puree for the sauce. Cook and stir over medium heat until mixture is reduced to a scant 1 cup (250 mL). Transfer to a bowl and chill for at least 30 minutes. Line a 9 × 5 in. (23 × 12.5-cm) loaf pan with plastic wrap. Transfer 1½ c. (375 mL) of the lemon sherbet to a large bowl. Fold in the reduced blackberry puree. Spread one-third of the remaining lemon sherbet in the bottom of the prepared loaf pan. Cover with the blackberry-lemon mixture. Top with the remaining lemon sherbet. Smooth the top and freeze overnight. When ready to serve, unmould parfait onto a decorative plate, allow to soften slightly, and pour reserved blackberry puree over the top. Slice into eight servings.

Yield: 8 servings
Exchange, 1 serving: ½ fruit
Calories, 1 serving: 27
Carbohydrates, 1 serving: 7 g

Chocolate Graham Cracker Ice-Cream Pie

| 1 qt. | reduced-calorie chocolate ice cream | 1 L |
| 1 c. | graham-cracker crumbs | 250 mL |

Slightly soften the ice cream. Spread half of the ice cream in the bottom of an 8-in. (20-cm) pie pan. Sprinkle half of the graham-cracker crumbs over the surface of the ice cream. (If mixture is very soft, you might want to place in freezer until surface is firm before continuing.) Spread remaining softened ice cream over the crumb top. Sprinkle with remaining graham-cracker crumbs. Freeze pie until firm. Cut into 12 wedges to serve.

Yield: 12 servings
Exchange, 1 serving: 1 bread
Calories, 1 serving: 82
Carbohydrates, 1 serving: 14 g

Frozen Raspberry Mousse with Black-Raspberry Sauce

2 pkgs. (4-serving)	sugar-free raspberry gelatin	2 pkgs. (4-serving)
2 c.	frozen black raspberries, slightly thawed	500 mL
¼ c.	water	60 mL
1 T.	cider vinegar	15 mL
1 stick	cinnamon	1 stick
1	egg white, beaten stiff	1
1 c.	prepared nondairy whipped topping	250 mL

Prepare both packages of raspberry gelatin together, as directed on package. Allow to completely set. Meanwhile, combine 1¼ c. (310 mL) of the black raspberries, water, cider vinegar, and cinnamon stick in a saucepan. Bring to a boil, reduce heat, and simmer for 5 to 6 minutes. If desired, strain mixture to remove seeds. Cool completely. Remove cinnamon stick. Beat the set raspberry gelatin with a wire whisk or electric mixer. Then beat ¼ c. (60 mL) of the black-raspberry sauce into the gelatin. Stir in the stiffly beaten egg white and the nondairy whipped topping. Spoon gelatin mixture into eight decorative glasses or bowls. Freeze until firm. To serve: Top frozen gelatin mixture with the remaining black-raspberry sauce. Garnish with the reserved ¾ c. (190 mL) of black raspberries.

Yield: 8 servings
Exchange, 1 serving: ⅓ fruit
Calories, 1 serving: 22
Carbohydrates, 1 serving: 4 g

Triple Sherbet Dessert

2 c.	reduced-calorie raspberry sherbet	500 mL
2 c.	reduced-calorie lemon sherbet	500 mL
2 c.	reduced-calorie lime sherbet	500 mL

Slightly soften raspberry sherbet. Spread into an 8-in. (20-cm) pie pan. Refreeze until firm. Slightly soften lemon sherbet. Spread over the surface of the raspberry sherbet. Refreeze. Slightly soften lime sherbet. Spread over the surface of the lemon sherbet. Refreeze until firm. Cut into 12 wedges to serve.

Yield: 12 servings
Exchange, 1 serving: ⅔ bread
Calories, 1 serving: 52
Carbohydrates, 1 serving: 9 g

Pink 'n' Pretty Strawberry Frozen Dessert

8-oz. box	sugar-free white cake mix	227-g box
1 pkg. (4-serving)	sugar-free strawberry gelatin	1 pkg. (4-serving)
1 c.	boiling water	250 mL
1 c.	frozen, unsweetened strawberries	250 mL
1	egg white, beaten stiff	1
¼ c.	prepared nondairy whipped topping	60 mL

Prepare cake mix as directed on package in a loaf pan. Cool in pan for 5 to 6 minutes. Move to rack and cool completely. Combine strawberry gelatin and boiling water in a mixing bowl. Stir to completely dissolve gelatin. Stir in strawberries. Allow to set. When gelatin has set, beat with an electric mixer. Stir in egg white and nondairy whipped topping. Chill until almost set. Cut cake into four layers. Divide the strawberry gelatin evenly among the layers and top. Freeze until firm (at least 6 hours). To serve: Heat a long knife in hot water, and wipe dry. Cut cake straight down (do not use a sawing back-and-forth motion). Clean knife between each serving.

Yield: 10 servings
Exchange, 1 serving: 1 bread
Calories, 1 serving: 105
Carbohydrates, 1 serving: 15 g

Ice-Cream Loaf with Raspberry Orange Sauce

1 qt.	reduced-calorie vanilla ice cream	1 L
12-oz. pkg.	frozen, unsweetened red raspberries	340-g pkg.
1 T.	all-natural apricot preserves	15 mL
⅓ c.	orange juice	90 mL
1 T.	lemon juice	15 mL
1⅓ c.	prepared nondairy whipped topping	340 mL
12	thinly sliced lemon-peel strips	12

Slightly soften ice cream. Line a 9 × 5 in. (23 × 12.5-cm) loaf pan with plastic wrap. Transfer softened ice cream to loaf pan. Freeze. Puree raspberries with the apricot preserves in a blender. If desired, strain to remove seeds. Add orange juice and lemon juice and stir to mix. Cover and refrigerate. To assemble: Unmould the ice cream onto a chilled platter. Spoon nondairy whipped topping into a pastry bag that has been fitted with a star tip. Pipe rosettes around base and 12 rosettes down middle of loaf of ice cream. Place a lemon strip on each of the middle rosettes. To serve: Spoon a small amount of raspberry orange sauce on one side of 12 chilled dessert plates. Cut ice-cream loaf into 12 slices. Place a slice of ice cream beside (not on top of) the raspberry orange sauce. Then drizzle the remaining sauce on each of the 12 slices.

Yield: 12 servings
Exchange, 1 serving: ⅔ bread, ⅓ fruit
Calories, 1 serving: 70
Carbohydrates, 1 serving: 15 g

Chocolate Ice-Cream Cake

8 in.	prepared sugar-free chocolate cake	23 cm
2½ c.	reduced-calorie chocolate ice cream	625 mL

Chill cake thoroughly. Cut cake in half horizontally. Slightly soften the ice cream. Spread 1 c. (250 mL) of the chocolate ice cream between the layers of the cake. Spread the remaining chocolate ice cream on the top of the cake. Freeze until firm. Allow cake to stand at room temperature for 10 minutes. Cut into 10 wedges to serve.

Yield: 10 servings
Exchange, 1 serving: 1½ bread, ½ fat
Calories, 1 serving: 150
Carbohydrates, 1 serving: 21 g

Luscious Lemon Ice-Cream Pie

1 qt.	reduced-calorie vanilla ice cream	1 L
1 pkg.	sugar-free lemon-pudding mix, prepared	1 pkg.
(4-serving)		(4-serving)

Slightly soften ice cream. Spread half of the ice cream on the bottom of an 8-in. (20-cm) pie pan. Spread half of the prepared lemon pudding on top of the ice cream. Spoon remaining ice cream over the top of the lemon pudding, spreading lightly. Spoon remaining lemon pudding over the top of the ice cream. Use a small knife to swirl the top pudding layer into the ice-cream layer below. Freeze until firm. Cut into 12 wedges to serve.

Yield: 12 servings
Exchange, 1 serving: ⅔ bread
Calories, 1 serving: 50
Carbohydrates, 1 serving: 9 g

Double-Decker Mocha Ice-Cream Pie

2 T.	instant coffee powder	30 mL
1 T.	boiling water	15 mL
1 qt.	reduced-calorie vanilla ice cream	1 L
8 in.	prepared chocolate pie crust	20 cm
1 qt.	reduced-calorie chocolate ice cream	1 L
1 c.	prepared nondairy whipped topping	250 mL

Dissolve the coffee powder in the boiling water. Allow to cool completely. Slightly soften the vanilla ice cream. Stir coffee liquid into vanilla ice cream. Freeze until almost firm. Spread coffee ice cream in the bottom of the chocolate crust. Slightly soften chocolate ice cream. Spread chocolate ice cream on top of coffee ice cream. Freeze until firm. Just before serving, spoon nondairy whipped topping into a pastry bag that has been fitted with a small star tip. Pipe rosettes decoratively on the top of the pie.

Yield: 8 servings
Exchange, 1 serving: 2 bread, ½ fat
Calories, 1 serving: 205
Carbohydrates, 1 serving: 29 g

Cakes

Cranberry Cake

2 c.	all-purpose flour	500 mL
½ c.	granulated sugar replacement	125 mL
¼ c.	granulated fructose	60 mL
2 t.	baking powder	10 mL
½ t.	salt	2 mL
1 c.	skim milk	250 mL
2	eggs	2
2 T.	solid shortening, softened	30 mL
2 t.	vanilla extract	10 mL
1½ c.	fresh cranberries	375 mL

Combine flour, sugar replacement, fructose, baking powder, and salt in a bowl. Add milk, eggs, shortening, and vanilla. Whisk or beat until smooth and creamy. Stir in cranberries. Transfer to a paper-lined or well-greased-and-floured 9-in. (23-cm)-square baking pan. Bake at 350 °F (175 °C) for 35 to 45 minutes or until pick inserted in middle comes out clean.

Yield: 16 servings
Exchange, 1 serving: 1 bread
Calories, 1 serving: 74
Carbohydrates, 1 serving: 13 g

Simple Cake

1⅓ c.	all-purpose flour	340 mL
½ c.	granulated sugar replacement	125 mL
1 T.	granulated fructose	15 mL
2 t.	baking powder	10 mL
⅔ c.	skim milk	180 mL

1	egg	1
2 T.	margarine, softened	30 mL
1 t.	vanilla extract	5 mL

Combine flour, sugar replacement, fructose, and baking powder in a food processor. Process on HIGH for 1 minute. Transfer dry ingredients to a medium-sized bowl. Add milk, egg, margarine, and vanilla. Beat on LOW for 30 seconds. Then beat on HIGH for 1 to 1½ minutes. Grease the bottom of an 8-in. (20-cm) round baking pan. (Do not grease the sides of the pan.) Line bottom with waxed paper and grease only the waxed paper. Transfer batter to prepared pan. Bake at 350 °F (175 °C) for 25 to 30 minutes or until pick inserted in middle comes out clean.

Yield: 10 servings
Exchange, 1 serving: 1 bread
Calories, 1 serving: 72
Carbohydrates, 1 serving: 13 g

Buttermilk Cake

1½ c.	sifted cake flour	375 mL
½ c.	granulated sugar replacement	125 mL
1 t.	baking powder	5 mL
½ t.	salt	2 mL
¼ t.	baking soda	1 mL
2 T.	solid shortening, softened	30 mL
¾ c.	buttermilk	190 mL
2	egg whites	2
1 t.	vanilla	5 mL

Sift together flour, sugar replacement, baking powder, salt, and baking soda into a medium-sized bowl. Add shortening and ½ c. (125 mL) of the buttermilk. Beat on MEDIUM for 2 minutes. Add remaining buttermilk, egg whites, and vanilla. Beat on HIGH for 2 minutes. Transfer batter into an 8-in. (20-cm) round well-greased-and-floured baking pan. Bake at 350 °F (175 °C) for 22 to 25 minutes or until pick inserted in middle comes out clean. Cool in pan for 5 minutes. Invert onto a cooling rack, and cool completely.

Yield: 10 servings
Exchange, 1 serving: 1 bread
Calories, 1 serving: 75
Carbohydrates, 1 serving: 12 g

Spice Raisin Cake

1⅓ c.	all-purpose flour	340 mL
½ c.	granulated sugar replacement	125 mL
1 T.	granulated fructose	15 mL
2 t.	baking powder	10 mL
1 t.	ground cinnamon	5 mL
¼ t.	ground nutmeg	1 mL
¼ t.	ground cloves	1 mL
¼ t.	ground ginger	1 mL
⅔ c.	skim milk	180 mL
1	egg	1
2 T.	margarine, softened	30 mL
1 t.	vanilla extract	5 mL
½ c.	plumped raisins	125 mL

Combine flour, sugar replacement, fructose, baking powder, cinnamon, nutmeg, cloves, and ginger in a medium-sized bowl. Add milk, egg, margarine, and vanilla. Beat on LOW for 30 seconds. Then beat on HIGH for 1 to 1½ minutes. Fold in raisins. Transfer batter to a well-greased-and-floured 9-in. (23-cm) round baking pan. Bake at 350 °F (175 °C) for 25 to 30 minutes or until pick inserted in middle comes out clean. (The all-purpose flour makes this cake a little heavy. If you prefer a lighter cake, sift the dry ingredients together several times before adding the liquid ingredients.)

Yield: 10 servings
Exchange, 1 serving: 1 bread, ⅓ fruit
Calories, 1 serving: 99
Carbohydrates, 1 serving: 17 g

Fructose Chocolate Cake

⅓ c.	granulated fructose	90 mL
1 c.	all-purpose flour	250 mL
¼ c.	unsweetened cocoa powder	60 mL
¾ t.	baking soda	4 mL
¼ t.	cream of tartar	1 mL
¼ c.	solid shortening, softened	60 mL
¾ c.	skim milk	190 mL

| 1 t. | vanilla extract | 5 mL |
| 1 | egg | 1 |

Place fructose in a small blender jar. Blend on HIGH for 20 seconds. (Fructose will powder.) Combine flour, fructose, cocoa, baking soda, and cream of tartar in a medium-sized bowl. Stir to mix. Add shortening, milk, and vanilla. Beat on LOW until blended. Then beat on HIGH for 1½ minutes. Add egg and continue beating on HIGH for 2 more minutes. Transfer batter to a greased-and-floured 8- or 9-in. (20- or 23-cm) round baking pan. Bake at 350 °F (175 °C) for 25 to 30 minutes or until pick inserted in middle comes out clean. Allow cake to cool in pan on cooling rack for 10 minutes. Remove from pan. Cool thoroughly on rack.

Yield: 10 servings
Exchange, 1 serving: 1 bread, 1 fat
Calories, 1 serving: 141
Carbohydrates, 1 serving: 16 g

Fructose White Cake

1⅓ c.	all-purpose flour	340 mL
¼ c.	granulated fructose	60 mL
2 t.	baking powder	10 mL
3 T.	margarine, softened	45 mL
⅔ c.	skim milk	180 mL
1	egg	1
1 t.	vanilla extract	5 mL

Combine flour, fructose, and baking powder in a food processor. Process on HIGH for 30 seconds. Add margarine and process for 30 seconds more. Transfer ingredients to a medium-sized bowl. Add milk, egg, and vanilla. Beat on LOW for 30 seconds. Then beat on HIGH for 2 minutes. Grease the bottom of an 8-in. (20-cm) round baking pan. (Do not grease the sides of the pan.) Line bottom with waxed paper and grease the waxed paper. Transfer batter to prepared pan. Bake at 350 °F (175 °C) for 25 to 30 minutes or until pick inserted in middle comes out clean.

Yield: 10 servings
Exchange, 1 serving: 1 bread, ½ fat
Calories, 1 serving: 109
Carbohydrates, 1 serving: 14 g

Perfect Chocolate Cake

8-oz. pkg.	fructose-sweetened chocolate cake mix	227-g pkg.
½ c.	water	125 mL
6	egg whites, room temperature	6

Line bottom of a 9-in. (23-cm) cake pan with waxed paper. (Do not grease bottom or sides of pan. Do not use a smaller cake pan; this cake will fill a 9-in. [23-cm] pan.) Combine cake mix and water in a mixing bowl. Beat on LOW just until mixed. Then beat on HIGH for 2 minutes. Add egg whites, and beat on HIGH for 5 to 7 minutes. Transfer cake batter to pan. Bake at 350 °F (175 °C) for 35 to 40 minutes or until pick inserted in middle comes out clean. Do not underbake. Allow cake to cool in pan for 10 minutes. Carefully slip a knife around the outside edge of the cake, invert to a cooling rack, and remove waxed paper. Invert to right-side-up position. Cool completely.

Yield: 10 servings
Exchange, 1 serving: 1 bread, ½ fat
Calories, 1 serving: 100
Carbohydrates, 1 serving: 18 g

Happy Birthday Cake

4.5-oz. box	sugar-free white frosting mix	128-g box
	food coloring	
1	prepared sugar-free cake	1
(10-serving)		(10-serving)
5	sugar-free hard candies	5
1 t.	sugar-free soft-drink mix powder	5 mL

Prepare frosting mix as directed on package. Set aside one-third of the frosting. Frost sides and top of cake. Tint the reserved frosting with food coloring. Using a small writing tip, pipe Happy Birthday on top of cake. Place hard candies (any color) in a heavy zip-lock plastic bag, and cover plastic bag with a folded washcloth. Using a hammer, pound the candies into small pieces. Sprinkle pieces around edges or over cake. Sprinkle soft-drink powder (any color) over cake.

Yield: 10 servings
Exchange, 1 serving: 1½ bread, ½ fat
Calories, 1 serving: 150
Carbohydrates, 1 serving: 24 g

Basket Cake

2 boxes (4.5-oz.)	sugar-free frosting mix	2 boxes (128-g)
8 in.	prepared round cake	20 cm
3 T.	unsweetened cocoa powder	45 mL
	green food coloring	
10	sugar-free gum drops	10

Prepare one box of frosting mix as directed on package. Frost sides and top of cake. Prepare second box of frosting mix as directed on package. Divide frosting in half and place in separate bowls. Add the cocoa to one of the bowls. Stir and blend completely. Using tip #21, pipe a medium-sized basket shape on top of the cake. Make a woven design or use loops or strips and wavy lines on the sides of the basket shape. Tint the second bowl of frosting green. Using various tips, make stems, leaves, and other designs emerging from the basket and/or around the cake. Cut gum drops lengthwise, fan, and place on stems for flowers.

Yield: 10 servings
Exchange, 1 serving: 1½ bread, ½ fat
Calories, 1 serving: 145
Carbohydrates, 1 serving: 22 g

Smiling Face

4.5-oz. box	sugar-free white frosting mix	128-g box
	yellow food coloring	
8 in.	prepared round cake	20 cm
6	sugar-free licorice gum drops	6

Prepare frosting mix as directed on package. Tint a bright yellow. Frost sides and top of cake. Cut licorice gum drops in half lengthwise. Place two halves in the position for an eye. Repeat for other eye. Cut one of the remaining halves in half widthwise. Place these two pieces in the middle for the nose. Place seven halves in the position for a smiling mouth.

Yield: 10 servings
Exchange, 1 serving: 1½ bread, ½ fat
Calories, 1 serving: 148
Carbohydrates, 1 serving: 23 g

Rainbow Cake

8 in.	prepared round sugar-free cake	20 cm
2 c.	prepared nondairy whipped topping	500 mL
	yellow food coloring	
	red food coloring	
	blue food coloring	

Frost the sides and top of the cake with a light coating of the white nondairy whipped topping. Use about one-third of the whipped topping. Transfer about ⅓ c. (90 mL) of white whipped topping to another small bowl. Tint yellow. Place the yellow whipped topping in the middle of the cake. Spread it into a circle to represent the sun. Spoon the remaining whipped topping equally into two small bowls. Tint one red, the other blue. Place and spread the red whipped topping in a semicircle around the "sun." Spread the blue whipped topping in a semicircle around the red whipped topping. The red and blue semicircles represent the rainbow.

Yield: 10 servings
Exchange, 1 serving: 1 bread, 1 fat
Calories, 1 serving: 136
Carbohydrates, 1 serving: 20 g

Butterfly Cake

8 in.	prepared round sugar-free cake	20 cm
4.5-oz. box	sugar-free white frosting mix	128-g box
	food coloring	
1 t.	sugar-free hot-cocoa mix powder	5 mL
12	sugar-free gum drops	12

Cut cake in half. Cut out a 1-in. (2.5-cm) equilateral triangle in the middle of the straight side of the cake. Place the cake on a decorative plate with the curved sides of the cake facing each other to form the body of the butterfly. Prepare frosting mix as directed on package. Use a very small amount of the white frosting to "stick" the two triangles together. Place it between the two pieces and at the top of the cake to form the head of the butterfly. Frost the head and the inside edges of the butterfly with the white frosting. Tint the remaining frosting a bright color, such as fuchsia, red, green, or aqua. Frost the outside edges of the butterfly with the bright frosting. Using the tips of a fork, draw across the top of the bright frosting into the white frosting to produce stripes. Sprinkle the cocoa powder on the head of the butterfly. Heat one gum drop at a time, either in your hand or in the microwave, for 5 to 6 seconds. Roll the gum drop with your fingers into a long round stripe. Repeat with five more gum drops. Arrange gum-drop stripes to radiate out from the middle of the curved edges of the butterfly body to the outside edges of the wings. Use six gum-drop stripes per side of butterfly.

Yield: 10 servings
Exchange, 1 serving: 1½ bread, ½ fat
Calories, 1 serving: 148
Carbohydrates, 1 serving: 23 g

Doll Cake

8-oz. pkg.	sugar-free cake mix	227-g pkg.
3 to 4 in.	plastic doll	7.5 to 10 cm
4.5-oz. box	sugar-free white frosting mix	128-g box
	food coloring	

Prepare cake mix as directed on package. Bake in a 1-qt. (1-L) half-circle metal gelatin mould or a plum-pudding mould. Baking time will be about 30 to 35 minutes, according to type of mould used. When a pick inserted in middle comes out clean, cake is done. (Middle will rise higher than sides.) Allow cake to cool in pan for 10 minutes; then move to rack to cool completely. Place cake on a decorative plate. Check height of doll to cake; cake should be to doll's waist or higher. Prepare white frosting mix as directed on package. Color, if desired. Place narrow strips of waxed paper around lower edge of cake. Frost the lower edge of the cake. Securely place the doll into the middle of the cake. Frost the top of the doll and then the skirt. Place a few drops of desired food coloring in a small bowl or glass. For lighter shades, add a few drops of water; for deep shades, use the coloring as is. With a small paint brush, color the dress of the doll. Always start with the lighter shades of color; then add deeper and darker color.

Yield: 10 servings
Exchange, 1 serving: 1½ bread, ½ fat
Calories, 1 serving: 147
Carbohydrates, 1 serving: 22 g

Ball Cake

4.5-oz. box	sugar-free white frosting mix	128-g box
8 in.	prepared round sugar-free cake	20 cm
10	sugar-free licorice gum drops	10
	food coloring	

Prepare frosting mix as directed on package. Frost sides and top of cake. Soften gum drops, one at a time, either in your hand or place in the microwave for 5 to 6 seconds. Roll gum drops with your fingers into a 4-in. (10-cm) strip. Place three strips down each side of the cake (in a curved design) to designate the stitching line. Cut remaining licorice strips into small pieces; place at an angle to the stitch line to finish the stitches. Place a few drops of food coloring (any color) in a small glass or bowl. With a small thin brush, write your message, such as the ball player's name, Great Game, or Congratulations.

Yield: 10 servings
Exchange, 1 serving: 1½ bread, ½ fat
Calories, 1 serving: 148
Carbohydrates, 1 serving: 23 g

Star Cake

8-oz. pkg.	sugar-free white cake mix	227-g pkg.
4.5-oz. box	sugar-free white frosting mix	128-g box
	blue food coloring	
	red food coloring	

Prepare cake mix as directed on package. Bake in a prepared 1-qt. (1-L) star-shaped gelatin mould. Allow cake to cool 10 minutes in pan before removing. Then cool completely. Prepare frosting mix as directed on package. Transfer one-third of the frosting to another bowl. Tint blue. Frost top third of the cake with the blue frosting. (This is one point and two half-points of the star form.) Transfer about one-third of the remaining white frosting to another bowl. Tint red. Make five stripes down the remaining part of the cake. Starting at the left side of the cake, frost first stripe white, second stripe red, continuing across cake.

Yield: 10 servings
Exchange, 1 serving: 1½ bread, ½ fat
Calories, 1 serving: 148
Carbohydrates, 1 serving: 23 g

Merry Christmas Wreath Cake

8-oz. pkg.	sugar-free cake mix	227-g pkg.
4.5-oz. box	sugar-free white frosting mix	128-g box
	green food coloring	
3	sugar-free red gum drops	3

Prepare cake mix as directed on package. Bake in a 1-qt. (1-L) shiny metal ring mould. Baking time will be about 20 to 25 minutes, according to type of mould used. When a pick inserted in middle comes out clean, cake is done. Allow cake to cool in pan for 10 minutes; then move to rack to cool completely. Prepare frosting mix as directed on package; tint a bright green. Frost cake. Soften gum drops one at a time, either in your hand or in the microwave for 5 to 6 seconds. Roll two of the gum drops with your fingers into a 4-in. (10-cm) strip. Roll the third gum drop into a 2-in. (5-cm) strip. Form the two 4-in. (10-cm) strips into the bow. Twist the 2-in. (5-cm) strip in the middle of the bow. Place in desired position on frosted cake.

Yield: 10 servings
Exchange, 1 serving: 1½ bread, ½ fat
Calories, 1 serving: 148
Carbohydrates, 1 serving: 23 g

Bell Cake

8 oz.	sugar-free white cake mix	227 g
4.5-oz. box	sugar-free white frosting mix	128-g box
	food coloring	

Prepare cake mix as directed on package, but bake in a bell-shaped pan. Allow to cool completely. Prepare frosting mix as directed on box. Frost the top and sides of the cake with a very light coating. Tint remaining frosting with color of your choice. Pipe designs on the cake, such as wedding bells or flowers, and messages, like Best Wishes or Happy New Year.

Yield: 10 servings
Exchange, 1 serving: 1½ bread, ½ fat
Calories, 1 serving: 143
Carbohydrates, 1 serving: 21 g

Cheesecakes

Lemon Cheesecake

Crust:

1 c.	saltine-cracker crumbs	250 mL
1 T.	soft margarine	15 mL
1 t.	grated lemon peel	5 mL

Filling:

1 pkg. (4-serving)	sugar-free lemon gelatin	1 pkg. (4-serving)
2 c.	hot water	500 mL
2 T.	finely grated lemon peel	30 mL
8-oz. pkg.	light cream cheese	227-g pkg.
1 c.	prepared nondairy whipped topping	250 mL

Crust: Mix together the saltine-cracker crumbs, margarine, and 1 t. (5 mL) of the lemon peel. Press into the bottom and slightly up the sides of an 8-in. (20-cm) pie pan. Refrigerate until ready to use.

Filling: Dissolve the lemon gelatin in the hot water. Stir in the 2 remaining T. (30 mL) of lemon peel, and allow to cool until mixture is a thick syrup. Whip cream cheese until light and fluffy. Gradually add lemon-gelatin mixture. Fold in nondairy whipped topping. Transfer to saltine-cracker crust. Refrigerate at least 2 to 3 hours or until firm.

Yield: 8 servings
Exchange, 1 serving: 1 bread, ¾ low-fat milk, 1 fat
Calories, 1 serving: 224
Carbohydrates, 1 serving: 23 g

Fresh Strawberry Cheesecake

Crust:

1½ c.	graham-cracker crumbs	375 mL
1 T.	soft margarine	15 mL
½ t.	ground nutmeg	2 mL
1 T.	water	5 mL

Filling:

8 oz.	low-fat cottage cheese	227 g
8-oz. pkg.	light cream cheese	227-g pkg.
⅔ c.	granulated sugar replacement	180 mL
1½ t.	vanilla extract	7 mL
2 env.	unflavored gelatin	2 env.
½ c.	cold water	125 mL
2 c.	prepared nondairy whipped topping	500 mL
3	egg whites, beaten stiff	3
2 c.	halved strawberries	500 mL

Crust: Mix the graham-cracker crumbs, margarine, and nutmeg together. Stir in the water until mixture is moist. Press into the bottom and slightly up the sides of a 10-in. (25-cm) springform pan. Refrigerate until ready to use.

Filling: Combine cottage cheese and cream cheese in a food processor or large bowl. Process or beat until cheeses are blended and creamy. Beat in sugar replacement and vanilla. Sprinkle and soften the gelatin in the cold water in a microwave-proof cup or bowl. Heat in the microwave for 1 to 2 minutes. Stir to dissolve the gelatin. Then completely fold the gelatin into the cheese mixture. Fold 1 c. (250 mL) of the prepared whipped topping and the three stiffly beaten egg whites into the cheese mixture. Transfer mixture to prepared crust. Chill thoroughly.

To serve: Remove sides of pan. Place cheesecake on decorative serving plate. Spread remaining 1 c. (250 mL) of nondairy whipped topping over top of cheesecake. Arrange the halved strawberries in the whipped topping.

Yield: 20 servings
Exchange, 1 serving: ¾ whole milk
Calories, 1 serving: 140
Carbohydrates, 1 serving: 9 g

Semisweet Chocolate Cheesecake

Crust:

1½ c.	vanilla-cookie crumbs	375 mL
1 T.	soft margarine	15 mL
1 T.	water	15 mL

Filling:

1 can (12-oz.)	skim evaporated milk	1 can (354-g)
2 T.	cornstarch	30 mL
⅛ t.	Stevia Rebaudiana extract	½ mL
	or	
⅓ c.	granulated fructose	90 mL
3 oz.	semisweet chocolate	86 g
2 pkgs. (8-oz.)	light cream cheese	2 pkgs. (227-g)
3	eggs	3
2 t.	chocolate extract	10 mL
1 t.	vanilla extract	5 mL
2 t.	all-purpose flour	10 mL

Crust: Combine crumbs, margarine, and water in a bowl or food processor. Blend completely. Press firmly into the bottom of a 9-in. (23-cm) springform pan. Refrigerate or place in freezer until chilled.

Filling: Combine evaporated milk, cornstarch, and sweetener of your choice in a saucepan. Cook and stir over medium heat until mixture is thick and very creamy. Remove from heat, add chocolate, and stir until chocolate is melted. Cool to room temperature. Beat cream cheese until light and fluffy. Beat in cooled chocolate-milk mixture. Beat in eggs, one at a time. Beat in chocolate and vanilla extracts and flour. Transfer to crumb-lined pan. Bake at 325 °F (165 °C) for 45 to 60 minutes or until middle is set. Allow to cool. Remove from pan. Chill thoroughly before serving.

Yield: 20 servings, with Stevia Rebaudiana
Exchange, 1 serving: ⅔ whole milk
Calories, 1 serving: 135
Carbohydrates, 1 serving: 9 g

Yield: 20 servings, with fructose
Exchange, 1 serving: 1 whole milk

Calories, 1 serving: 148
Carbohydrates, 1 serving: 12 g

Cherry Cheesecake

Crust:

1½ c.	cornflake crumbs	375 mL
1 T.	soft margarine	15 mL
½ t.	liquid Stevia Rebaudiana extract (page 8)	2 mL
1 t.	water	5 mL

Filling:

8-oz. pkg.	light cream cheese	227-g pkg.
1 T.	liquid Stevia Rebaudiana extract (page 8)	15 mL
2	eggs, separated	2
1½ T.	all-purpose flour	21 mL
⅛ t.	salt	½ mL
½ t.	vanilla extract	2 mL
½ c.	evaporated milk, chilled	125 mL
1½ T.	lemon juice	21 mL

Topping:

1½ c.	fresh tart red cherries	375 mL
½ c.	water	125 mL
1 T.	liquid Stevia Rebaudiana extract (page 8)	15 mL
1 env.	unflavored gelatin	1 env.
2 T.	cold water	30 mL
	red food coloring	

Crust: Mix together cornflake crumbs, margarine, and the ½ t. (2 mL) of Stevia Rebaudiana liquid. Add the 1 t. (5 mL) of water and thoroughly blend. Press into bottom and slightly up sides of a 9-in. (23-cm) spring-form pan. Refrigerate until ready to use.

Filling: Whip the cream cheese until soft and fluffy. Beat in 1 T. (15 mL) of Stevia Rebaudiana liquid and egg yolks (one at a time). Beat in the flour, salt, and vanilla extract. Whip the evaporated milk until thick, add the lemon juice, and continue beating until stiff. Gently fold into cream mixture. Beat the egg whites until stiff. Fold into the cream mixture. Transfer to prepared cornflake crust. Bake at 325 °F (165 °C) for 1 hour. Turn off heat and allow cheesecake to cool in oven.

Topping: Combine tart cherries, the ½ c. (125 mL) of water, and the 1 T. (15 mL) of Stevia Rebaudiana liquid in a saucepan. Mix well and bring to a boil. Reduce heat and simmer for 8 minutes. Dissolve the gelatin in 2 T. (30 mL) of cold water. Stir into cherry mixture. Cook until gelatin is dissolved. Remove from heat. Add a few drops of red food coloring. Cool until thickened. At serving time, spread cherry mixture over cheesecake.

Yield: 20 servings
Exchange, 1 serving: 1 bread, 1 fat
Calories, 1 serving: 125
Carbohydrates, 1 serving: 15 g

Cinnamon Apple Cheesecake

Crust:

1 c.	graham-cracker crumbs	250 mL
1 T.	soft margarine	15 mL
1 t.	ground cinnamon	5 mL

Filling:

2 c.	cinnamon apple juice	500 mL
1 env.	unflavored gelatin	1 env.
1 pkg.	sugar-free vanilla pudding	1 pkg.
(4-serving)	mix (to cook)	(4-serving)
3 in.	cinnamon stick	7.5 cm
8-oz. pkg.	light cream cheese	227-g pkg.

Crust: Mix together the graham-cracker crumbs, margarine, and cinnamon. Press into the bottom and slightly up the sides of an 8-in. (20-cm) pie pan. Refrigerate until ready to use.

Filling: Pour cinnamon apple juice in a saucepan. Sprinkle gelatin over top and allow to soften for 3 to 4 minutes. Stir in pudding mix. Add cinnamon stick. Cook and stir over medium heat until mixture is smooth and thickened. Remove from heat and allow to cool to room temperature.

Remove cinnamon after mixture is cooled. Whip cream cheese until light and fluffy. Slowly add cooled cinnamon-apple mixture. Beat thoroughly. Pour into 8-in. (20-cm) graham-cracker crust. Refrigerate at least 2 to 3 hours or until firm.

Yield: 8 servings
Exchange, 1 serving: 1 bread, 1 low-fat milk, 1 fat
Calories, 1 serving: 240
Carbohydrates, 1 serving: 26 g

Sweet Breads

Chocolate Cinnamon Rolls

½ c.	skim milk	125 mL
1 pkg.	dry yeast	1 pkg
¼ c.	warm water	1 mL
⅔ c.	granulated sugar replacement	180 mL
	or	
⅛ t.	Stevia Rebaudiana extract	½ mL
¼ c.	solid shortening	60 mL
1 T.	granulated fructose	15 mL
1	egg	1
½ t.	salt	2 mL
⅓ c.	unsweetened baking cocoa	90 mL
2½ c.	all-purpose flour	625 mL
2 T.	margarine, melted	30 mL
3 T.	granulated sugar replacement	45 mL
2 t.	ground cinnamon	10 mL

Pour skim milk in small saucepan. Bring to a boil, remove from heat, and allow to cool. Dissolve the yeast in the warm water. Combine skim milk, yeast mixture, sweetener of your choice, fructose, shortening, egg, and salt in a large mixing bowl. Combine the cocoa with 1¼ c. (310 mL) of flour in another bowl. Stir to mix. Add to liquid mixture in bowl. Beat on LOW until mixture is blended and smooth. Add remaining flour and stir until all the flour is incorporated into the dough. Turn out onto a lightly floured surface; then knead for 4 to 5 minutes until dough is smooth and elastic. Place in a greased bowl, turn dough over, cover, and allow to rise until double in size (about 1½ hours). Punch dough down and roll into a 12 × 9 in. (30 × 23 cm) rectangle. Spread with melted margarine. Combine the 3 T. (45 mL) sugar replacement and cinnamon in a bowl. Stir to mix. Sprinkle over surface of dough. Roll up, beginning at the 12-in. (30-cm) side. Tuck end of dough into the roll to seal. Cut into 18 slices. Place slices slightly apart in a 13 × 9 in. (33 × 23 cm) well-greased pan. Cover, and allow to rise until double in size (about 45 to 60 minutes). Bake at 375 °F (190 °C) for 25 to 30 minutes or until done.

Yield: 18 servings
Exchange, 1 serving: ¾ bread
Calories, 1 serving: 60
Carbohydrates, 1 serving: 11 g

Cherry Coffee Cake

1 pkg.	dry yeast	1 pkg.
¼ c.	warm water	60 mL
¾ c.	skim milk	190 mL
1 T.	cider vinegar	15 mL
½ c.	granulated sugar replacement	125 mL
2 T.	margarine, softened	30 mL
1	egg	1
1 t.	baking powder	5 mL
½ t.	salt	2 mL
3¼ c.	all-purpose flour	810 mL
1½ c.	fresh or frozen sweet cherries, thawed and drained	375 mL

Dissolve yeast in warm water in a large mixing bowl. Add milk, vinegar, sugar replacement, margarine, egg, baking powder, salt, and 2 c. (500 mL) of the flour. Beat on LOW until mixture is blended; then mix on MEDIUM for 2 minutes. Stir in remaining flour. Transfer to a lightly floured surface, and knead until smooth and elastic (about 5 minutes). Roll dough into a 20 × 6 in. (50 × 15 cm) rectangle. Place on a greased cookie sheet. Cut 2-in. (5-cm) slices on each of the 20-in. (50-cm) sides of the dough. Cut cherries in quarters. Place cherries lengthwise down the middle of the rectangles. Crisscross sliced strips over cherries. Cover and allow to rise in a warm place until double in size. Bake at 375 °F (190 °C) for 20 to 22 minutes or until golden brown.

Yield: 22 servings
Exchange, 1 serving: ¾ bread
Calories, 1 serving: 63
Carbohydrates, 1 serving: 13 g

Cherry Chocolate Coffee Cake

2 c.	frozen, unsweetened sweet cherries	500 mL
1½ t.	cornstarch	7 mL
¼ t.	unsweetened black-cherry soft-drink mix powder	1 mL
¼ t.	ground nutmeg	1 mL
½ c.	skim milk	125 mL
1 pkg.	dry yeast	1 pkg.
¼ c.	warm water	1 mL
⅔ c.	granulated sugar replacement	180 mL
	or	
⅛ t.	Stevia Rebaudiana extract	½ mL
¼ c.	solid shortening	60 mL
1	egg	1
½ t.	salt	2 mL
⅓ c.	unsweetened baking cocoa	90 mL
2½ c.	all-purpose flour	625 mL
2 T.	margarine, melted	30 mL

Place frozen cherries in a 1-qt. (1-L) microwave measuring cup. Heat in microwave on MEDIUM for 2 minutes. Stir and then continue heating on MEDIUM for another 2 minutes. Cherries should be thawed but not hot. Use a scissors to cut cherries into pieces. (If cherries are hot, allow to cool before stirring in cornstarch.) Stir in cornstarch, soft-drink mix powder, and nutmeg. Place back in microwave and cook for 3 to 4 minutes on MEDIUM-HIGH or until mixture is very thick and clear. Set aside to cool completely. Meanwhile, pour skim milk in small saucepan. Bring to a boil, remove from heat, and allow to cool. Dissolve the yeast in the warm water. Combine skim milk, yeast mixture, sweetener of your choice, shortening, egg, and salt in a large mixing bowl. Combine the cocoa with 1¼ c. (310 mL) of flour in another bowl. Stir to mix. Add to liquid mixture in bowl. Beat on LOW until mixture is blended and smooth. Add remaining flour and stir until all the flour is incorporated into the dough. Turn out onto a lightly floured surface; then knead for 4 to 5 minutes until dough is smooth and elastic. Place in a greased bowl, turn dough over, cover, and allow to rise until double in size (about 1½ hours). Punch dough down and roll into a 25 × 12 in. (62 × 30 cm) rectangle. Place dough on a well-greased cookie sheet. Make 3-in. (7.5-cm) diagonal cuts at 1-in. (2.5-cm) intervals on the 25-in. (62-cm) side of the rectangle with a scissors. Spread cherry filling down the middle of the coffee-cake dough. Crisscross cut strips at an angle over filling, overlapping the strips so that they are about 1 in. (2.5-cm) apart. Cover coffee cake with plastic wrap, then a towel. Allow to rise until double in size (about 45 to 60 minutes). Bake at 350 °F (175 °C) for 25 to 30 minutes or until done. While warm, brush with melted margarine.

Yield: 18 servings
Exchange, 1 serving: ¾ bread
Calories, 1 serving: 62
Carbohydrates, 1 serving: 12 g

Easy Apple Coffee Cake

1-lb. loaf	frozen bread dough, thawed	500-g loaf
2 T.	margarine, melted	30 mL
¼ c.	granulated brown-sugar replacement	60 mL
1 T.	all-purpose flour	15 mL
2 t.	ground cinnamon	10 mL
1 t.	ground nutmeg	5 mL
2 c.	grated peeled apple	500 mL

Divide bread dough in half. Roll each half into an 8-in. (20-cm) square. Place each square on a greased cookie sheet. Brush with melted margarine. Combine brown-sugar replacement, flour, cinnamon, and nutmeg in a bowl. Stir to mix. Add grated apple and toss to coat apple. Spoon one-half of the apple mixture down the middle of each square. Cut 2-in. (5-cm) strips down two of the sides, towards the apple filling, about 1 in. (2.5 cm) apart. Fold strips alternately, overlapping the filling. Cover and allow coffee cake to rise until double in size. Bake at 350 °F (175 °C) for 30 to 35 minutes or until golden brown.

Yield: 32 servings
Exchange, 1 serving: ½ bread, ¼ fruit
Calories, 1 serving: 57
Carbohydrates, 1 serving: 12 g

Tart Orange Coffee Cake

1 pkg.	dry yeast	1 pkg.
¼ c.	warm water	60 mL
12-oz. can	frozen orange-juice concentrate, slightly thawed	355-mL can
1	egg	1
½ t.	salt	2 mL
2 c.	all-purpose flour	500 mL
1 T.	solid shortening, melted	15 mL
1 T.	cornstarch	15 mL
2 T.	cold water	30 mL
1 t.	vanilla extract	5 mL

Dissolve the yeast in warm water. Allow to rest for 5 minutes. Pour into medium-sized mixing bowl. Heat ½ c. (125 mL) of the orange-juice concentrate just until the chill is off. Pour into yeast mixture. Add egg, salt, and 1 c. (250 mL) of the flour. Beat on LOW to blend. Then beat on HIGH for 2 minutes. Stir in remaining 1 c. (250 mL) of flour. Beat on LOW for 1 minute (dough will be soft). Brush about two-thirds of the melted shortening on bottom and sides of a medium-sized bowl. Transfer dough to greased bowl. Brush remaining melted shortening on top of dough. Cover with plastic wrap and then a towel. Allow to rise until double in size. Meanwhile, dissolve cornstarch in cold water. Pour into a saucepan. Add remaining orange-juice concentrate. Stir to mix. Cook and stir over medium heat until mixture is very thick. Remove from heat and stir in vanilla. Allow to cool completely. To assemble: Flour your hands and divide dough in half. Press one-half of the dough into the bottom of a greased 9-in. (23-cm) round springform pan, pressing slightly up the sides. Spoon about one-half of the orange-juice mixture over the top. Transfer remaining half of dough to a floured surface. Press to flatten dough to a 9-in. (23-cm) round. Place dough round on top of orange-juice mixture in pan. Make random indentations in the top of the dough. Spoon remaining orange-juice mixture over top. Allow to rise uncovered for 30 to 40 minutes. Place in cold oven. Set oven for 350 °F (175 °C). Bake for 25 to 30 minutes or until done. Allow coffee cake to cool in pan 10 minutes; then release sides.

Yield: 18 servings
Exchange, 1 serving: ¾ bread
Calories, 1 serving: 66
Carbohydrates, 1 serving: 14 g

Chocolate Raised Doughnuts

½ c.	skim milk	125 mL
1 pkg.	dry yeast	1 pkg.
¼ c.	warm water	1 mL
⅔ c.	granulated sugar replacement	180 mL
	or	
⅛ t.	Stevia Rebaudiana extract	½ mL
¼ c.	solid shortening	60 mL
2 T.	granulated fructose	30 mL
1	egg	1
½ t.	salt	2 mL
⅓ c.	unsweetened baking cocoa	90 mL
2½ c.	all-purpose flour	625 mL

Pour skim milk in small saucepan. Bring to a boil, remove from heat, and allow to cool. Dissolve the yeast in the warm water. Combine skim milk, yeast mixture, sweetener of your choice, shortening, fructose, egg, and salt in a large mixing bowl. Combine the cocoa with 1¼ c. (310 mL) of flour in another bowl. Stir to mix. Add to liquid mixture in bowl. Beat on LOW until mixture is blended and smooth. Add remaining flour and stir until all the flour is incorporated into the dough. Turn out onto a lightly floured surface; then knead for 4 to 5 minutes or until dough is smooth and elastic. Place in a greased bowl, turn dough over, cover, and allow to rise until double in size (about 1½ hours). Punch dough down and roll to about ½ in. (1.25 cm) thickness. Cut with floured doughnut cutter. Place doughnuts onto a greased cookie sheet or piece of waxed paper. Cover and allow to rise. Heat 2 to 3 in. (5 to 8 cm) of oil in deep-fat fryer or heavy saucepan to 375 °F (190 °C). Heat a wide spatula in the oil. Gently slide spatula under a doughnut. Place doughnut in the hot oil, and fry about 2 minutes on each side. Remove from oil; drain on paper towels. Repeat with remaining doughnuts.

Yield: 18 servings
Exchange, 1 serving: ¾ bread
Calories, 1 serving: 65
Carbohydrates, 1 serving: 14 g

Buttermilk Doughnuts

1 pkg.	dry yeast	1 pkg.	
¼ c.	warm water	60 mL	
1 c.	buttermilk, warmed	250 mL	
1	egg	1	
½ t.	salt	2 mL	
2 T.	margarine, melted	30 mL	
½ c.	granulated sugar replacement	125 mL	
1 T.	granulated fructose	15 mL	
3 c.	all-purpose flour	750 mL	

Dissolve yeast in warm water. Allow to rest for 5 minutes; then pour into a large mixing bowl. Add buttermilk, egg, salt, margarine, sugar replacement, fructose, and 2 c. (500 mL) of the flour. Beat on LOW until blended. Then beat on HIGH for 2 minutes. Stir in remaining 1 c. (250 mL) of flour. Transfer dough to a floured surface. Knead until smooth and elastic. Transfer to a greased bowl; turn dough over. Cover with plastic wrap and then a towel. Allow to rise until double in size. Transfer to a lightly floured surface. Pat or roll dough to about ⅓-in. (8-mm) thickness. Cut with floured doughnut cutter. Allow to rest for 10 to 15 minutes. Heat about 3 in. (7.5 cm) of vegetable oil to 375 °F (190 °C) in a skillet or deep-fat fryer. Slide doughnuts into hot oil. Fry until golden brown, turning several times. Remove from oil and drain on paper towels.

Yield: 24 servings
Exchange, 1 serving: ¾ bread
Calories, 1 serving: 63
Carbohydrates, 1 serving: 13 g

Dutch Doughnuts

1 pkg.	dry yeast	1 pkg.	
¼ c.	warm water	60 mL	
2	eggs	2	
½ c.	skim milk	125 mL	
¼ c.	whole milk	60 mL	
1 t.	vanilla extract	5 mL	
⅓ c.	granulated sugar replacement	90 mL	
3 c.	all-purpose flour	750 mL	
1 T.	baking powder	15 mL	
1 t.	salt	5 mL	

| ½ t. | ground cinnamon | 2 mL |
| ¼ t. | ground nutmeg | 1 mL |

Dissolve yeast in warm water in a large bowl. Add eggs, skim and whole milk, vanilla, and sugar replacement. Beat until light and fluffy. Add 2 c. (500 mL) of the flour and the baking powder, salt, cinnamon, and nutmeg; beat on LOW until well blended. Stir in remaining flour. Transfer to floured surface. Roll dough to about ⅓-in. (8-mm) thickness. Cut with a floured doughnut cutter. Heat about 3 in. (7.5 cm) of vegetable oil to 375 °F (190 °C) in a skillet or deep-fat fryer. Slide doughnuts into hot oil. Fry until golden brown, turning several times. Remove from oil and drain on paper towels.

Yield: 24 servings
Exchange, 1 serving: ¾ bread
Calories, 1 serving: 60
Carbohydrates, 1 serving: 12 g

Cinnamon Swirl Bread

1-lb. loaf	frozen bread dough, thawed	500-g loaf
1 T.	margarine, melted	15 mL
⅛ t.	Stevia Rebaudiana extract	½ mL
(scant)		(scant)
	or	
⅓ c.	granulated sugar replacement	90 mL
1 T.	ground cinnamon	15 mL

Roll dough into a 12 × 7 in. (30 × 17 cm) rectangle. If using Stevia Rebaudiana, dissolve it in the melted margarine, spread dough surface with the melted-margarine mixture, and sprinkle with the cinnamon. If using sugar replacement, spread dough with melted margarine, mix the sugar replacement with the cinnamon, and sprinkle mixture on top of dough. Roll up jelly roll–style, starting from the short end. Seal edges and end of loaf. Place, seam side down, in a greased loaf pan. Allow to rise. Bake at 375 °F (190 °C) for 25 to 30 minutes or until done. Remove from oven. Remove loaf from pan. Cool.

Yield: 18 servings
Exchange, 1 serving: ¾ bread
Calories, 1 serving: 58
Carbohydrates, 1 serving: 15 g

Cinnamon Rolls

Dough mixture:

½ c.	skim milk	125 mL
2 t.	cider vinegar	10 mL
1 pkg.	dry yeast	1 pkg.
¼ c.	warm water	60 mL
⅓ c.	granulated sugar replacement	90 mL
	or	
2 t.	granulated fructose	10 mL
3 T.	solid shortening	45 mL
1	egg	1
½ t.	salt	2 mL
3 c.	all-purpose flour	750 mL

Cinnamon mixture:

1 T.	margarine, melted	15 mL
⅛ t. (scant)	Stevia Rebaudiana extract	½ mL (scant)
	or	
⅓ c.	granulated sugar replacement	90 mL
	ground cinnamon	

Dough: Combine skim milk and vinegar in a large mixing bowl. Dissolve the yeast in the warm water. Add to skim-milk mixture. Beat in sweetener of your choice, shortening, egg, and salt. Next, add 2 c. (500 mL) of the flour. Beat on LOW until the mixture is blended and smooth. Then add remaining flour and stir until all the flour is incorporated into the dough. Turn out onto a lightly floured surface; knead for 4 to 5 minutes until dough is smooth and elastic. Place in a greased bowl, turn dough over, cover, and allow to rise until double in size (about 1½ hours). Punch dough down and roll into a 12 × 9 in. (30 × 23 cm) rectangle.

Cinnamon mixture: If using Stevia Rebaudiana, dissolve it in the melted margarine, spread dough surface with the melted-margarine mixture, and sprinkle with desired amount of cinnamon. If using sugar replacement, spread dough with melted margarine, mix the sugar replacement with desired amount of cinnamon, and sprinkle mixture on top of dough.

To assemble: Roll up, beginning at the 12-in. (30-cm) side. Tuck end of dough into the roll to seal. Cut into 18 slices. Place slightly apart in a 13 × 9 in. (33 × 23 cm) well-greased pan. Cover, and allow to rise until double in size (about 45 to 60 minutes). Bake at 375 °F (190 °C) for 25 to 30 minutes or until done.

Yield: 18 servings
Exchange, 1 serving: 1 bread
Calories, 1 serving: 73
Carbohydrates, 1 serving: 13 g

Pecan Rolls

1 pkg.	dry yeast	1 pkg.
¼ c.	warm water	60 mL
½ c.	whole milk	125 mL
2 T.	margarine, softened	30 mL
½ c.	granulated sugar replacement	125 mL
	or	
3 T.	granulated fructose	45 mL
1	egg	1
½ t.	salt	2 mL
2½ c.	all-purpose flour	625 mL
1 T.	margarine, melted	15 mL
⅛ t.	Stevia Rebaudiana extract	½ mL
(scant)		(scant)
	or	
⅓ c.	granulated sugar replacement	90 mL
	ground cinnamon	
½ c.	sugar-free maple-flavored syrup	125 mL
⅓ c.	ground pecans	90 mL

Dissolve the yeast in the warm water. Allow to rest for 2 minutes. Pour into a large mixing bowl. Add milk, softened margarine, the ½ c. of sugar replacement or the 3 T. of fructose, egg, salt, and 1½ c. (375 mL) of the flour. Beat on LOW to blend, then on HIGH for 2 minutes. Stir in remaining 1 c. (250 mL) of flour. Transfer to a lightly floured surface; knead until smooth and elastic. Place in a greased bowl, turn dough over, and cover with plastic wrap and then a towel. Allow to rise until double in size. Punch dough down and roll into a 12 × 9 in. (30 × 23 cm) rectangle. If using Stevia Rebaudiana, dissolve it in the melted margarine, spread dough surface with the melted-margarine mixture, and sprinkle with desired amount of cinnamon. If using sugar replacement, spread dough with melted margarine, mix the sugar replacement with desired amount of cinnamon, and sprinkle mixture on top of dough. To assemble: Roll up, beginning at the 12-in. (30-cm) side. Tuck end of dough into the roll to seal. Cut into 18 slices. Pour sugar-free maple-flavored syrup in the bottom of a well-greased 13 × 9 in. (33 × 23 cm) pan. Sprinkle pecans over surface of syrup. Place slices of dough on top of the pecans. Then cover, and allow to rise until double in size (about 45 to 60 minutes). Bake at 375 °F (190 °C) for 25 to 30 minutes or until done.

Yield: 18 servings
Exchange, 1 serving: 1 bread
Calories, 1 serving: 78
Carbohydrates, 1 serving: 16 g

Buttermilk Sticky Rolls

1 pkg.	dry yeast	1 pkg.
¼ c.	warm water	60 mL
¾ c.	buttermilk	190 mL
2 T.	margarine, softened	30 mL
½ c.	granulated sugar replacement	125 mL
	or	
3 T.	granulated fructose	45 mL
1	egg	1
½ t.	salt	2 mL
3 c.	all-purpose flour	750 mL
1 T.	margarine, melted	15 mL
⅛ t.	Stevia Rebaudiana extract	½ mL
(scant)		(scant)
	or	
⅓ c.	granulated sugar replacement	90 mL
	ground cinnamon	
½ c.	sugar-free maple-flavored syrup	125 mL

Dissolve the yeast in the warm water. Allow to rest for 2 minutes. Pour into a large mixing bowl. Add buttermilk, softened margarine, sweetener of your choice, egg, salt, and 2 c. (500 mL) of the flour. Beat on LOW to blend, then on HIGH for 2 minutes. Stir in remaining 1 c. (250 mL) of flour. Transfer to a lightly floured surface, and knead until smooth and elastic. Place in a greased bowl, turn dough over, and cover with plastic wrap and then a towel. Allow to rise until double in size. Punch dough down and roll into a 12 × 9 in. (30 × 23 cm) rectangle. If using Stevia Rebaudiana, dissolve it in the melted margarine, spread dough surface with the melted-margarine mixture, and sprinkle with desired amount of cinnamon. If using sugar replacement, spread dough with melted margarine, mix the sugar replacement with desired amount of cinnamon, and sprinkle mixture on top of dough.

To assemble: Roll up, beginning at the 12-in. (30-cm) side. Tuck end of dough into the roll to seal. Cut into 18 slices. Pour sugar-free maple-flavored syrup in the bottom of a well-greased 13 × 9 in. (33 × 23 cm) pan. Place the cut slices of dough slightly apart on top of the syrup. Cover, and allow to rise until double in size (about 45 to 60 minutes). Bake at 375 °F (190 °C) for 25 to 30 minutes or until done.

Yield: 18 servings
Exchange, 1 serving: 1 bread
Calories, 1 serving: 72
Carbohydrates, 1 serving: 12 g

Braided Raisin Bread

| 1-lb. loaf | frozen bread dough, thawed | 500-g loaf |
| 1 c. | raisins, cut in half | 250 mL |

With your hands, work the raisins into the dough. Divide the dough into three pieces. Cover and allow to rest for 10 minutes. Roll each piece of dough into a ball. Then roll each ball into a rope about 16 in. (40 cm) long. Line up the three dough ropes, about 1 in. (2.5 cm) apart on a greased baking sheet. Very loosely braid the ropes. (Braid by bringing outside ropes alternately over middle rope.) Allow to rise. Bake at 375 °F (190 °C) for 25 to 30 minutes or until done.

Yield: 18 servings
Exchange, 1 serving: 1 bread, 1/3 fruit
Calories, 1 serving: 81
Carbohydrates, 1 serving: 19 g

Quick Breads

Pumpkin Bread

2 c.	all-purpose flour	500 mL
1 c.	granulated brown-sugar replacement	250 mL
1 T.	baking powder	15 mL
2 t.	ground cinnamon	10 mL
½ t.	ground nutmeg	2 mL
¼ t.	salt	1 mL
¼ t.	baking soda	1 mL
⅛ t.	ground cloves	½ mL
1 c.	canned pumpkin	250 mL
½ c.	skim milk	125 mL
2	eggs	2
⅓ c.	solid shortening	90 mL

Combine 1 c. (250 mL) of the flour and the brown-sugar replacement, baking powder, cinnamon, nutmeg, salt, baking soda, and cloves in a large mixing bowl. Add the remaining flour, pumpkin, milk, eggs, and shortening. Beat with an electric mixer on LOW until mixed. Then beat on HIGH for 1 to 2 minutes until well blended. Grease a 9 × 5 × 3 in. (23 × 13 × 8 cm)-loaf pan on the bottom and ½ in. (1.25 cm) up the sides. Transfer batter to pan. Bake at 350 °F (175 °C) for 60 to 65 minutes or until pick inserted in middle comes out clean. Cool in pan for 10 minutes. Carefully slip a knife around the edge of the bread. Transfer to a cooling rack. Allow to cool. Wrap cooled bread in plastic wrap and store at room temperature for a day before slicing.

Yield: 20 servings
Exchange, 1 serving: 1 bread
Calories, 1 serving: 85
Carbohydrates, 1 serving: 15 g

Quick Blueberry Nut Muffins

2 c.	biscuit mix	500 mL
¼ c.	granulated sugar replacement	60 mL
¾ c.	skim milk	190 mL
2 T.	margarine, melted	30 mL
1 c.	fresh or frozen blueberries	250 mL
⅓ c.	walnuts, chopped	90 mL

Combine biscuit mix, sugar replacement, milk, and margarine in a medium-sized mixing bowl. Stir to mix. (Batter will be lumpy.) Stir in fresh or frozen blueberries and nuts. Line 12 large muffin cups with paper liners. Divide batter evenly among the muffin cups. Bake at 400 °F (200 °C) for 20 to 25 minutes or until pick inserted in muffin comes out clean.

Yield: 12 servings
Exchange, 1 serving: 1⅓ bread
Calories, 1 serving: 112
Carbohydrates, 1 serving: 20 g

Sweet Corn Cake

1 c.	all-purpose flour	250 mL
¾ c.	cornmeal	190 mL
1 T.	baking powder	15 mL
½ t.	salt	2 mL
1 c.	skim milk	250 mL
1	egg, beaten	1
2 T.	liquid fructose	30 mL
2 T.	margarine, melted	30 mL

Sift together flour, cornmeal, baking powder, and salt into a bowl. In a large mixing bowl, combine milk, egg, fructose, and margarine. Beat with a fork to blend. Stir flour mixture into milk mixture, just enough to moisten. Transfer batter into a greased 8-in. (20-cm) round baking pan. Bake at 400 °F (200 °C) for 30 to 35 minutes or until pick inserted in middle comes out clean.

Yield: 12 servings
Exchange, 1 serving: 1 bread
Calories, 1 serving: 99
Carbohydrates, 1 serving: 16 g

Banana Bread

1¾ c.	all-purpose flour	440 mL
1 T.	granulated fructose	15 mL
⅛ t.	Stevia Rebaudiana extract	½ mL
2 t.	baking powder	10 mL
½ t.	baking soda	2 mL
¼ t.	salt	1 mL
1 c.	mashed banana	250 mL
⅓ c.	solid shortening	90 mL
2 T.	skim milk	30 mL
2	eggs	2

Combine 1 c. (250 mL) of the flour and the fructose, Stevia Rebaudiana, baking powder, baking soda, and salt in a large mixing bowl. Add banana, shortening, and milk. Then add remaining flour. Beat until well blended (at least 2 minutes). Add eggs, one at a time, beating well after each addition. Transfer batter to a well-greased 8 × 4 × 2 in. (20 × 10 × 5 cm)-loaf pan. Bake at 350 °F (175 °C) for 55 to 65 minutes or until pick inserted in middle comes out clean. Remove from oven, and allow to cool in pan 10 minutes. Transfer to cooling rack. This bread is best the second day.

Yield: 16 servings
Exchange, 1 serving: 1 bread
Calories, 1 serving: 87
Carbohydrates, 1 serving: 17 g

Rhubarb Nut Bread

2 c.	frozen rhubarb	500 mL
2 c.	all-purpose flour	500 mL
1 t.	baking soda	5 mL
½ t.	cream of tartar	2 mL
½ t.	salt	2 mL
⅔ c.	granulated sugar replacement	180 mL
	or	
⅛ t.	Stevia Rebaudiana extract	½ mL
3 T.	granulated fructose	45 mL
⅓ c.	hot water	90 mL
1	egg	1

| 2 T. | vegetable oil | 30 mL |
| ⅓ c. | walnuts, chopped | 90 mL |

Chop frozen rhubarb very small, or place frozen rhubarb in food processor and process until chopped. (Rhubarb will have an icy appearance.) Set aside. Combine flour, baking soda, cream of tartar, salt, sweetener of your choice, fructose, hot water, egg, and vegetable oil in a mixing bowl. Beat to blend. Add frozen rhubarb. Beat to mix. Beat in nuts. Batter will be very stiff. Allow batter to set for 10 minutes. Beat slightly. Grease two 5 × 3 × 2 in. (13 × 8 × 5 cm)-loaf pans on the bottom and about ½ in. (1.25 cm) up the sides. Spoon batter evenly between the two pans. Bake at 350 °F (175 °C) for 50 to 55 minutes. Allow bread to cool in pans for 10 minutes. Carefully slip a knife around the edge of the bread. Transfer to a cooling rack. Allow to cool. Wrap cooled bread in plastic wrap and store at room temperature for a day before slicing.

Yield: 24 servings
Exchange, 1 serving: ¾ bread
Calories, 1 serving: 48
Carbohydrates, 1 serving: 12 g

Pineapple Oatmeal Coffee Cake

1 c.	quick-cooking oatmeal	250 mL
1 c.	unsweetened pineapple juice	250 mL
2 t.	baking powder	10 mL
½ t.	baking soda	2 mL
1	egg	1
1 c.	all-purpose flour	250 mL
3 env.	aspartame sweetener	3 env.

Combine oatmeal and pineapple juice in a mixing bowl. Stir to mix. Allow to rest for 10 to 15 minutes. Add baking powder, baking soda, and egg. Stir vigorously with a spoon. Then stir in flour. Transfer to a greased 9-in. (23-cm) round baking pan. Bake at 350 °F (175 °C) for 25 to 35 minutes or until pick inserted in middle comes out clean. Remove from oven. Sprinkle top with aspartame sweetener.

Yield: 16 servings
Exchange, 1 serving: ¾ bread
Calories, 1 serving: 66
Carbohydrates, 1 serving: 12 g

Sweet Zucchini Bread

1 c.	grated, unpeeled zucchini	250 mL
1 c.	granulated sugar replacement	250 mL
	or	
⅛ t.	Stevia Rebaudiana extract	½ mL
¼ c.	vegetable oil	60 mL
1	egg, slightly beaten	1
¼ t.	grated lemon peel	1 mL
1½ c.	all-purpose flour	375 mL
2 T.	granulated fructose	30 mL
1 t.	ground cinnamon	5 mL
1 t.	baking soda	5 mL
½ t.	cream of tartar	2 mL
¼ t.	ground nutmeg	1 mL
⅛ t.	ground allspice	½ mL

Combine zucchini, sweetener of your choice, oil, egg, and lemon peel in a large mixing bowl. Stir to mix. Combine flour, fructose, cinnamon, baking soda, cream of tartar, nutmeg, and allspice in another bowl. Stir to mix. Add flour mixture to zucchini mixture. Stir just enough to blend. Transfer batter to a well-greased 8 × 4 × 2 in. (20 × 10 × 5 cm)-loaf pan. Bake at 350 °F (175 °C) for 55 to 65 minutes or until pick inserted in middle comes out clean. Remove from oven, and allow to cool in pan 10 minutes. Transfer to cooling rack. This bread is best the second day.

Yield: 16 servings
Exchange, 1 serving: 1 bread
Calories, 1 serving: 82
Carbohydrates, 1 serving: 15 g

Apricot-Jam Muffins

1 c.	quick-cooking oatmeal	250 mL
1 c.	buttermilk	250 mL
1	egg	1
2 T.	margarine, softened	30 mL
1 c.	all-purpose flour	250 mL
⅓ c.	granulated sugar replacement	90 mL
2 T.	granulated fructose	30 mL
2 t.	baking powder	10 mL
1 t.	baking soda	5 mL

½ t.	salt	2 mL
6 t.	all-natural apricot preserves	30 mL

Combine oatmeal and buttermilk in a large mixing bowl. Stir to blend. Allow to rest for 10 minutes. Stir in egg and margarine. Stir in flour, sugar replacement, fructose, baking powder, baking soda, and salt until well blended. Line 12 large muffin cups with paper liners. Divide batter evenly among the muffin cups. Top each muffin with ½ t. (2 mL) of the apricot preserves. Bake at 350 °F (175 °C) for 20 to 25 minutes or until pick inserted in muffin comes out clean.

Yield: 12 servings
Exchange, 1 serving: 1 bread
Calories, 1 serving: 99
Carbohydrates, 1 serving: 17 g

Oatmeal Walnut Muffins

1 c.	quick-cooking oatmeal	250 mL
1 c.	buttermilk	250 mL
1	egg	1
2 T.	margarine, softened	30 mL
1 c.	all-purpose flour	250 mL
⅓ c.	granulated sugar replacement	90 mL
2 T.	granulated fructose	30 mL
2 t.	baking powder	10 mL
1 t.	baking soda	5 mL
½ t.	salt	2 mL
⅓ c.	walnuts, chopped fine	90 mL

Combine oatmeal and buttermilk in a large mixing bowl. Stir to blend. Allow to rest for 10 minutes. Stir in egg and margarine. Stir in flour, sugar replacement, fructose, baking powder, baking soda, and salt until well blended. Then stir in the walnuts. Allow batter to rest for 2 minutes. Line 12 large muffin cups with paper liners. Divide batter evenly among the muffin cups. Bake at 375 °F (190 °C) for 20 to 25 minutes or until pick inserted in muffin comes out clean.

Yield: 12 servings
Exchange, 1 serving: 1⅓ bread
Calories, 1 serving: 121
Carbohydrates, 1 serving: 19 g

Cranberry Muffins

1¼ c.	all-purpose flour	310 mL
¼ c.	whole-wheat flour	60 mL
½ c.	yellow cornmeal	125 mL
½ c.	granulated sugar replacement	125 mL
1 T.	granulated fructose	15 mL
1 T.	baking powder	15 mL
1 t.	baking soda	5 mL
1 t.	ground cinnamon	5 mL
dash	salt	dash
1¼ c.	buttermilk	310 mL
1 c.	fresh cranberries, chopped	250 mL
1	egg	1
1	egg white	1
3 T.	vegetable oil	45 mL

Combine flours, cornmeal, sugar replacement, fructose, baking powder, baking soda, cinnamon, and salt in a large mixing bowl. Stir to mix. Add buttermilk, cranberries, egg, egg white, and oil. Beat to blend. Line 12 muffin cups with paper cups. Divide the batter evenly among the cups. Bake at 425 °F (220 °C) for 20 minutes or until muffins are golden brown. Transfer to cooling rack and cool slightly. Serve warm.

Yield: 12 servings
Exchange, 1 serving: 1⅓ bread
Calories, 1 serving: 110
Carbohydrates, 1 serving: 20 g

Strawberry Banana Muffins

2 c.	biscuit mix	500 mL
¼ c.	granulated sugar replacement	60 mL
¾ c.	skim milk	190 mL
2 T.	margarine, melted	30 mL
12 medium	fresh strawberries	12 medium
2 small	bananas	2 small

Combine biscuit mix, sugar replacement, milk, and margarine in a medium-sized mixing bowl. Stir to mix. (Batter will be lumpy.) Cut strawberries and bananas into small cube-like pieces. Stir into batter. Line 12 large muffin cups with paper liners. Divide batter evenly among the muffin cups. Bake at 400 °F (200 °C) for 20 to 25 minutes or until pick inserted in muffin comes out clean.

Yield: 12 servings
Exchange, 1 serving: 1⅓ bread
Calories, 1 serving: 112
Carbohydrates, 1 serving: 19 g

Big Sweet Biscuits

3 c.	all-purpose flour	750 mL
3 T.	granulated sugar replacement	45 mL
1 T.	granulated fructose	15 mL
4 t.	baking powder	20 mL
¾ t.	cream of tartar	4 mL
½ t.	salt	2 mL
¼ t.	baking soda	1 mL
¾ c.	solid shortening, softened	190 mL
1	egg, beaten	1
1 c.	skim milk	250 mL

Combine flour, sugar replacement, fructose, baking powder, cream of tartar, salt, and baking soda in a large mixing bowl. Cut in shortening with a pastry cutter or knives until mixture becomes coarse crumbs. (This part can also be done in a food processor.) Combine egg and milk. Stir into flour mixture just enough to make a soft dough. Transfer dough to a floured surface. Knead lightly 10 to 15 times. Pat or roll out to about 1-in. (2.5-cm) thickness. Cut 16 biscuits with a floured 2-in. (5-cm) dough-nut cutter. Place on ungreased cookie sheet. Bake at 450 °F (230 °C) for 12 to 15 minutes or until golden brown. They are best if served immediately.

Yield: 16 servings
Exchange, 1 serving: 2 bread
Calories, 1 serving: 163
Carbohydrates, 1 serving: 28 g

Pancakes, Waffles & Crepes

Cinnamon Apple Raisin Dessert Pancakes

1½ c.	all-purpose flour	375 mL
¼ c.	granulated sugar replacement	60 mL
	or	
2 T.	granulated fructose	30 mL
	or	
2 t.	liquid Stevia Rebaudiana extract (page 8)	10 mL
2 t.	baking powder	10 mL
½ t.	salt	2 mL
½ t.	ground allspice	2 mL
½ t.	ground cinnamon	2 mL
1¼ c.	skim milk, room temperature	310 mL
2	eggs	2
3 T.	margarine, melted	45 mL
½ t.	vanilla extract	2 mL
1-lb. can	unsweetened apple slices	454-g can
½ c.	raisins	125 mL
¾ t.	ground cinnamon	4 mL
3 env.	aspartame sweetener	3 env.

Combine flour, sweetener of your choice, baking powder, salt, allspice, and the ½ t. (2 mL) of cinnamon in a bowl. Whisk together 1 c. (250 mL) of the milk and the eggs, melted margarine, and vanilla. Stir liquid into dry mixture just until blended. Cover and refrigerate at least 1 hour. Combine apple slices, raisins, and the ¾ t. (4 mL) of cinnamon in a bowl. Stir to blend. To assemble: Stir remaining ¼ c. (60 mL) of milk into the pancake batter. Heat a griddle or heavy large skillet over medium-high heat; spray with a vegetable oil. Ladle batter onto griddle, using about ½ c. (125 mL) of batter. Top with about 2 T. (30 mL) of the apple-raisin mixture. Then fry until bubbles appear on the surface. Flip pancake and cook until bottom is golden brown. Transfer to a heated platter. Repeat procedure with remaining batter. To serve: Place pancakes on dessert plates, apple side up. Divide any remaining apple mixture among the pancakes. Sprinkle each pancake with one-fourth envelope of aspartame sweetener.

Yield: 12 servings, with granulated sugar replacement or liquid Stevia
    Rebaudiana
Exchange, 1 serving: ½ bread, 1 fruit, ¼ fat
Calories, 1 serving: 123
Carbohydrates, 1 serving: 21 g

Yield: 12 servings, with granulated fructose
Exchange, 1 serving: ½ bread, 1 fruit, ¼ fat
Calories, 1 serving: 128
Carbohydrates, 1 serving: 21 g

Apricot Dessert Cakes with Apricot Sauce

1-lb. can	apricots in juice	454-g can
1 c.	biscuit mix	250 mL
4 env.	aspartame sweetener	4 env.
4 T.	prepared nondairy whipped topping	60 mL

Drain apricot juice from apricots into a measuring cup. Add enough water to make ¾-c. liquid. Combine apricot juice and biscuit mix in a bowl. Beat until well blended. Heat a griddle or nonstick skillet over medium heat; spray with a vegetable oil. Ladle about one-fourth of the batter onto the greased surface. Fry until bubbles begin to appear on surface. Turn over and fry until bottom is golden brown. Transfer to warmed platter. Repeat procedure with remaining batter. Transfer apricots to a food processor or blender. Process to a puree. Pour apricot puree into a small sauce pan. Heat thoroughly. Remove from heat and stir in aspartame sweetener. To serve: Place each apricot pancake on a dessert plate. Divide the warm apricot puree evenly among the pancakes. Top each pancake with 1 T. (15 mL) of the nondairy whipped topping. Serve immediately.

Yield: 4 servings
Exchange, 1 serving: ½ bread, ½ fruit
Calories, 1 serving: 65
Carbohydrates, 1 serving: 14 g

Blueberry Ricotta Sweet Pancakes

4	eggs, separated	4
1 c.	ricotta cheese made from skim milk	250 mL
1/3 c.	nonfat plain yogurt	90 mL
3 T.	granulated sugar replacement	45 mL
	or	
1½ T.	granulated fructose	21 mL
2/3 c.	all-purpose flour	180 mL
2 t.	baking powder	10 mL
dash	salt	dash
3/4 c.	skim milk	190 mL
2 c.	fresh blueberries	500 mL
1 c.	prepared nondairy whipped topping	250 mL

Combine egg yolks, ricotta cheese, yogurt, and sweetener of your choice in a bowl. Beat to blend thoroughly. Sift flour, baking powder, and salt together. Stir into cheese mixture. Stir in milk. Fold in blueberries. Beat egg whites until stiff. Fold into batter. Heat a griddle or heavy nonstick skillet over medium heat; spray with a vegetable oil. Ladle about 3 T. (45 mL) of batter onto greased surface. Fry until bubbles begin to appear on surface. Turn over and fry until bottom is golden brown. Transfer to warmed platter. Repeat procedure with remaining batter. To serve: Roll each pancake into a tube. Pipe nondairy whipped topping over pancakes.

Yield: 20 servings, with granulated sugar replacement
Exchange, 1 serving: 1 bread
Calories, 1 serving: 75
Carbohydrates, 1 serving: 14 g

Yield: 20 servings, with granulated fructose
Exchange, 1 serving: ½ bread
Calories, 1 serving: 76
Carbohydrates, 1 serving: 14 g

Sweet Cakes with Warm Maple-Cinnamon Topping

1 2/3 c.	nonfat milk	430 mL
1	egg	1
3 T.	liquid fructose	45 mL
2 T.	vegetable oil	30 mL
1 t.	vanilla extract	5 mL

1 c.	all-purpose flour	250 mL
½ c.	whole-wheat flour	125 mL
2 T.	yellow cornmeal	30 mL
1 T.	oat bran	15 mL
1 t.	baking powder	5 mL
1 t.	ground cinnamon	5 mL
¼ t.	salt	1 mL
½ c.	sugar-free maple-flavored syrup	125 mL
½ t.	ground cinnamon	2 mL

Combine milk, egg, fructose, vegetable oil, and vanilla in a bowl. Beat to blend. Combine flours, cornmeal, oat bran, baking powder, the 1 t. (5 mL) of cinnamon, and the salt in large bowl. Stir to mix. Gradually pour the milk mixture into the flour mixture, stirring or beating on LOW constantly until the batter is smooth. Heat a griddle or nonstick skillet over medium heat. Grease lightly with a vegetable spray. Spoon batter, about 2 T. (30 mL) at a time, onto the hot griddle. Fry until golden brown on the bottom; turn and fry on the other side. Transfer to warmed platter. Repeat procedure with remaining batter. Combine maple-flavored syrup and the ½ t. (2 mL) of cinnamon in a small saucepan or microwave bowl. Stir over medium heat until warmed. To serve: Place pancakes on decorative warmed platter, passing maple-cinnamon topping separately.

Yield: 16 servings
Exchange, 1 serving: ¾ bread
Calories, 1 serving: 65
Carbohydrates, 1 serving: 11 g

Kids-Kolored Kakes

2 c.	biscuit mix	500 mL
2 t.	unsweetened soft-drink mix (flavor and color of your choice)	10 mL
1¼ c.	skim milk	310 mL

Combine all ingredients in a bowl. Beat to blend. Fry as directed on biscuit package.

Yield: 16 servings
Exchange, 1 serving: ⅔ bread
Calories, 1 serving: 62
Carbohydrates, 1 serving: 11 g

German Apple Pancake

3 large	eggs	3 large
⅔ c.	whole milk	180 mL
½ c.	all-purpose flour	125 mL
¼ c.	margarine, melted	60 mL
¼ c.	granulated sugar replacement	60 mL
1 t.	ground cinnamon	5 mL
1 large	green apple (peeled, halved, cored, and cut into very thin slices)	1 large

Place eggs, whole milk, flour, 2 T. (30 mL) of the melted margarine, 1 T. (15 mL) of the sugar replacement, and ½ t. (2 mL) of the cinnamon in a bowl or food processor. Beat or process until well blended and smooth. Set aside. Brush remaining melted margarine over bottom and sides of a 10-in. (25-cm) heavy oven-proof skillet or pan. Add apple slices, and sprinkle with remaining sugar replacement and cinnamon. Place on top of stove and cook over medium heat until apple slices are tender. Remove from heat, and arrange apple slices in a single layer in the bottom of the same skillet. Pour batter over apple slices, and bake at 450 °F (230 °C) for 15 minutes or until golden brown. Remove from oven. Cut around outside edge of pancake, and invert on warmed decorative dessert platter. Cut into four wedges and serve immediately.

Yield: 4 servings
Exchange, 1 serving: ⅔ bread, ½ fruit, 2 fat
Calories, 1 serving: 155
Carbohydrates, 1 serving: 17 g

Strawberries and Cream Waffles

2 c.	fresh or frozen unsweetened strawberries, thawed	500 mL
5 env.	aspartame sweetener	5 env.
¼ c.	liquid nondairy creamer	60 mL
½ c.	prepared nondairy whipped topping	125 mL
6	frozen waffles, thawed and toasted	6

Place strawberries in a bowl; mash slightly with a fork. Sprinkle with aspartame sweetener and stir. Add nondairy creamer. Mix thoroughly. Fold in nondairy whipped topping. To serve: Place hot waffles on dessert plates. Divide the strawberry cream evenly among the waffles. Serve immediately.

Yield: 6 servings
Exchange, 1 serving: 1 bread, ½ fat
Calories, 1 serving: 125
Carbohydrates, 1 serving: 14 g

Pumpkin Waffles

1½ c.	all-purpose flour	375 mL
2 t.	baking powder	10 mL
¾ t.	ground cinnamon	4 mL
½ t.	baking soda	2 mL
¼ t.	salt	1 mL
¼ t.	ground cloves	1 mL
1¼ c.	buttermilk	310 mL
¾ c.	pumpkin puree	190 mL
2	eggs, separated	2
2 T.	sugar-free maple-flavored syrup	30 mL
2 t.	vegetable oil	10 mL
2 c.	low-calorie vanilla ice cream	500 mL

Combine flour, baking powder, cinnamon, baking soda, salt, and cloves in a bowl. Stir to mix. In another bowl, combine buttermilk, pumpkin puree, egg yolks, maple-flavored syrup, and vegetable oil. Beat until well blended. Add pumpkin mixture to flour mixture. Fold and stir until flour mixture is moistened. Beat egg whites until stiff. Carefully fold egg whites into pumpkin batter. Do not overmix. Heat a waffle iron according to manufacturer's directions. Grease the iron lightly with a vegetable spray. Spoon the batter onto the iron, filling the surface to about two-thirds full. (Use amount of batter to make total of four large or eight small waffles.) Close the lid and cook for 5 to 6 minutes or until golden brown. Transfer to heated platter. Repeat procedure with remaining batter. To serve: Slice or break large waffles in half. Place waffle-half on a warmed plate. Divide the ice cream evenly among the eight waffle servings. Swirl ice cream in a circular pattern around the top of the waffle. Serve immediately.

Yield: 8 servings
Exchange, 1 serving: 1½ bread
Calories, 1 serving: 130
Carbohydrates, 1 serving: 21 g

Basic Crepes

1¼ c.	all-purpose flour	310 mL
dash	salt	dash
3	eggs, beaten	3
1½ c.	skim milk	375 mL
2 T.	vegetable oil	30 mL
2 T.	granulated sugar replacement	30 mL
	or	
2 t.	granulated fructose	10 mL

Place all ingredients in a blender, food processor, or bowl. Process batter thoroughly. Cover, refrigerate, and allow batter to rest 1 to 24 hours. To fry: Batter should be the consistency of light cream. If necessary, add a small amount of water to batter. Heat an 8-in. (20-cm) nonstick skillet or crepe iron over medium heat until a drop of water sizzles when sprinkled on the surface. Reduce heat a little. Use crepe iron as directed by manufacturer. Spray nonstick skillet with a vegetable-oil spray. Remove skillet from heat. Spoon in 2 T. (30 mL) of batter. Tilt skillet in a circle to spread batter around bottom. Return to heat, and brown crepe on one side. Invert pan over a plate or paper towel. Repeat using remaining batter.

Yield: 20 crepes
Exchange, 1 crepe: ⅔ bread
Calories, 1 crepe: 50
Carbohydrates, 1 crepe: 5 g

Chocolate Crepes

¼ c.	skim milk	60 mL
6 T.	all-purpose flour	90 mL
2 T.	unsweetened cocoa powder	30 mL
dash	salt	dash
1 t.	granulated fructose	5 mL
1	egg	1
2 t.	vegetable oil	10 mL

Combine all ingredients in order given in a blender or bowl. Beat until blended and smooth. Cover, and refrigerate 1 to 24 hours. To fry: Batter should be the consistency of light cream. If necessary, add a small amount of water to batter. Heat an 8-in. (20-cm) nonstick skillet or crepe iron over medium heat until a drop of water sizzles when sprinkled on the surface. Reduce heat a little. Use crepe iron as directed by manufacturer. Spray nonstick skillet with a vegetable-oil spray. Remove skillet from heat. Spoon in 2 T. (30 mL) of batter. Tilt skillet in a circle to spread batter around bottom. Return to heat, and brown crepe on one side. Invert pan over a plate or paper towel. Repeat using remaining batter.

Yield: 8 crepes
Exchange, 1 crepe: ⅔ bread
Calories, 1 crepe: 50
Carbohydrates, 1 crepe: 5 g

Chocolate Crepes with Chocolate and Orange Sauce

1 c.	ricotta cheese made with skim milk	250 mL
1 t.	vanilla extract	5 mL
1 T.	boiling water	15 mL
1 T.	all-natural orange marmalade	15 mL
3 T.	unsweetened cocoa powder	45 mL
1½ t.	cornstarch	7 mL
1½ t.	granulated sugar replacement	7 mL
3 T.	skim milk	45 mL
1 T.	liquid fructose	15 mL
½ t.	vegetable oil	2 mL
½ t.	vanilla extract	2 mL
6 env.	aspartame sweetener	6 env.
8	prepared Chocolate Crepes (opposite page)	8

Combine ricotta cheese and the 1 t. (5 mL) of vanilla in a bowl. Stir to blend thoroughly. Set aside. Combine boiling water and orange marmalade in a small cup or bowl. Stir to dissolve jam. Set aside. Combine cocoa powder, cornstarch, and sugar replacement in a saucepan. Gradually stir in the milk and fructose. Bring to a boil, continually stirring. Reduce heat and simmer on LOW 1 to 2 minutes or until thickened. Remove from heat, and stir in vegetable oil, the ½ t. (2 mL) of vanilla, and aspartame sweetener. Set aside. To assemble: Lay each crepe on a decorative plate. Spread the ricotta mixture evenly down the middle of the crepes. Roll crepes up jelly roll–style. Spoon 1 T. (15 mL) of the chocolate sauce over each crepe. Then spoon the orange sauce over the crepes. Serve immediately.

Yield: 8 servings
Exchange, 1 serving: ⅔ bread, ⅓ low-fat milk
Calories, 1 serving: 89
Carbohydrates, 1 serving: 9 g

Chocolate Crepes with Pistachio Cream and Raspberries

1 pkg. (4-serving)	sugar-free instant pistachio pudding mix	1 pkg. (4-serving)
1	egg white	1
½ c.	prepared nondairy whipped topping	125 mL
8	Chocolate Crepes (page 82)	8
32	fresh ripe raspberries	32

Prepare pistachio pudding mix as directed on package. Set until firm. Beat egg white until stiff. Fold a small amount of egg white into pistachio pudding to loosen. Fold pudding into egg white. Carefully fold in non-dairy whipped topping. To assemble: Place crepes on dessert plates. Fill one-half of each crepe with pistachio filling. Fold crepe in half, covering the pistachio filling. Lay four raspberries next to each crepe.

Yield: 8 servings
Exchange, 1 serving: 1 bread
Calories, 1 serving: 100
Carbohydrates, 1 serving: 14 g

Blueberry Crepes with Vanilla-Pudding Sauce

1 qt.	fresh blueberries	1 L
8 env.	aspartame sweetener	8 env.
1 pkg. (4-serving)	sugar-free instant vanilla-pudding mix	1 pkg. (4-serving)
2½ c.	skim milk	625 mL
20	Basic Crepes (page 82)	20

Clean and lightly crush blueberries. Stir in aspartame sweetener and set aside. Combine vanilla pudding and milk in a bowl. Blend with a wire whisk or electric beater on LOW until well blended. Set aside. Divide the blueberry mixture evenly among the crepes. Fold each crepe in half and place in a large decorative dessert dish. Pour vanilla pudding over the crepes. Refrigerate at least 2 hours before serving.

Yield: 20 servings
Exchange, 1 serving: ¾ bread
Calories, 1 serving: 65
Carbohydrates, 1 serving: 7 g

Apple Crepes

3 lbs.	Golden Delicious apples	1½ Kg
¾ c.	granulated sugar replacement	190 mL
¾ c.	water	190 mL
1 T.	lemon juice	15 mL
1 t.	rum flavoring	5 mL
⅛ t.	ground cinnamon	½ mL
½ t.	ground nutmeg	2 mL
1 c.	water	250 mL
1 t.	cornstarch	5 ml.
1 T.	cold water	15 mL
4 env.	aspartame sweetener	4 env.
12	Basic Crepes (page 82)	12

Peel apples and reserve peel. Core and thinly slice apples. Combine apple slices, sugar replacement, and the ¾ c. (190 mL) of water, lemon juice, rum flavoring, cinnamon, and nutmeg in a nonstick saucepan. Bring to a boil, reduce heat, and simmer until apples are tender. Stir frequently. Set aside. Combine apple peels and the 1 c. (250 mL) of water in another saucepan. Bring to a boil, reduce heat, and simmer until peels are tender. Transfer the apple peels and the liquid to a blender or food processor. Process to a puree. Strain back into saucepan. Dissolve cornstarch in the 1 T. (15 mL) of cold water. Stir into the pureed apple-peel liquid. Return to heat, and cook and stir until mixture is clear and beginning to thicken. When mixture has cooled, stir in aspartame sweetener. To assemble: Divide apple-slice mixture evenly among the 12 crepes. Roll up jelly-roll style. Lay seam side down in a lightly greased baking dish. Cover with foil and bake at 350 °F (175 °C) for 10 minutes or until crepes are heated through. Transfer crepes to warmed platter Warm apple-peel sauce just slightly. Transfer to a warmed sauce dish. Serve crepes, passing the warm sauce separately.

Yield: 12 servings
Exchange, 1 serving: ⅔ bread, 1 fruit
Calories, 1 serving: 102
Carbohydrates, 1 serving: 18 g

Pies

Pastry Shell (from Mix)

| 1 | pie-crust stick or mix, for a 9-in. (23-cm) shell | 1 |

Prepare dough as directed on package. Form dough into a 9-in. (23-cm) microwave or glass pie pan. Trim and flute edges as desired. Prick bottom and sides of unbaked shell. Microwave on MEDIUM HIGH for 4 to 5 minutes. Rotate dish one-fourth turn after 2 minutes, then again in 2 minutes. Cool.

Yield: 8 servings
Exchange, 1 serving: 1 bread, 1 fat
Calories, 1 serving: 123
Carbohydrates, 1 serving: 15 g

Graham-Cracker Crust

| ⅓ c. | reduced-calorie margarine | 90 mL |
| 1½ c. | graham-cracker crumbs | 375 mL |

Melt margarine in a 9-in. (23-cm) microwave or glass pie dish. Add cracker crumbs. Using a fork, completely blend crumbs and margarine. Press evenly onto bottom and sides of dish. Microwave, uncovered, on HIGH for 2 minutes. Rotate dish one-fourth turn after 1 minute. Allow crust to rest and cool before filling.

Yield: 8 servings
Exchange, 1 serving: 1 bread, 1 fat
Calories, 1 serving: 120
Carbohydrates, 1 serving: 16 g

Wafer Crust

| ⅓ c. | reduced-calorie margarine | 90 mL |
| 1½ c. | wafer crumbs (vanilla or chocolate) | 375 mL |

Melt margarine in a 9-in. (23-cm) microwave or glass pie dish. Add wafer crumbs. Using a fork, completely blend crumbs and margarine. Press evenly onto bottom and sides of dish. Microwave, uncovered, on HIGH for 2 minutes. Rotate dish one-fourth turn after 1 minute. Allow crust to rest and cool before filling.

Yield: 8 servings, with vanilla crumbs
Exchange, 1 serving: 1 bread, 1 fat
Calories, 1 serving: 120
Carbohydrates, 1 serving: 15 g

Yield: 8 servings, with chocolate crumbs
Exchange, 1 serving: 1 bread, 1 fat
Calories, 1 serving: 130
Carbohydrates, 1 serving: 18 g

Flaky Pie Crust (Two Shells)

1½ c.	all-purpose flour	375 mL
dash	salt	dash
½ c.	solid vegetable shortening	125 mL
1	egg	1
1 t.	white vinegar	5 mL
2 T.	water	30 mL
2 to 3 drops	yellow food coloring	2 to 3 drops

Sift flour, measure, and resift into a bowl or food processor. Add salt and shortening. Using a pastry blender or food processor, cut until mixture becomes coarse crumbs. In a small bowl, combine egg, vinegar, water, and food coloring. Lightly beat to blend. Drizzle into flour mixture, mixing lightly until all the flour is moistened and forms into a ball. Divide the dough in half, roll out each piece on a lightly floured board, and fit into two 9-in. (23-cm) microwave or glass pie dishes. Prick bottom and sides of each shell. Microwave each shell on MEDIUM HIGH for 4 to 5 minutes. Rotate dish one-fourth turn after 2 minutes, then again in 2 minutes. Cool.

Yield: 8 servings/shells
Exchange, 1 serving: 1 bread, 3 fat
Calories, 1 serving: 214
Carbohydrates, 1 serving: 16 g

Meringue Pie Shell

3	egg whites	3
½ t.	vanilla extract	2 mL
¼ t.	cream of tartar	1 mL
dash	salt	dash
½ c.	granulated sugar replacement	125 mL
	or	
⅛ t.	Stevia Rebaudiana extract	½ mL
(scant)		(scant)

Combine egg whites, vanilla, cream of tartar, and salt in a bowl. Beat to soft peaks. Gradually beat in sugar replacement or add Stevia Rebaudiana extract. Beat to stiff peaks. Spread on the bottom and sides of a 9-in. (23-cm) pie pan. Bake at 300 °F (150 °C) for 35 to 40 minutes or until crisp and lightly browned. Cool completely before using.

Yield: 8 servings
Exchange, 1 serving: negligible
Calories, 1 serving: negligible
Carbohydrates, 1 serving: negligible

Nut Meringue Pie Shell

3	egg whites	3
½ t.	vanilla extract	2 mL
¼ t.	cream of tartar	1 mL
dash	salt	dash
½ c.	granulated sugar replacement	125 mL
¼ c.	chopped nuts	60 mL

Combine egg whites, vanilla, cream of tartar, and salt in a bowl. Beat to soft peaks. Gradually beat in sugar replacement. Beat to stiff peaks. Spread on the bottom and sides of a 9-in. (23-cm) pie pan. Sprinkle with chopped nuts. Bake at 275 °F (135 °C) for 1 hour. Cool completely before using.

Yield: 8 servings
Exchange, 1 serving: ½ fat
Calories, 1 serving: 23
Carbohydrates, 1 serving: negligible

Chocolate-Chip Pie

1 recipe	Nut Meringue Pie Shell (opposite page)	1 recipe
½ c.	semisweet chocolate chips	125 mL
¼ c.	hot water	60 mL
1 t.	vanilla extract	5 mL
dash	salt	dash
2 c.	prepared nondairy whipped topping	500 mL

Melt chocolate chips in the top of a double boiler over simmering water. Stir in hot water, vanilla, and salt. Stir and cook until smooth. Cool completely. Fold in nondairy whipped topping. Transfer to prepared pie shell. Chill at least 5 hours or overnight.

Yield: 8 servings
Exchange, 1 serving: ¾ bread, ¾ fat
Calories, 1 serving: 92
Carbohydrates, 1 serving: 9 g

Sweet Cherry Dessert Pie

10 in.	baked pie shell	25 cm
1-lb. bag	frozen, unsweetened sweet cherries, thawed	457-g bag
1 env.	unflavored gelatin	1 env.
¼ c.	cold water	60 mL
2 c.	prepared nondairy whipped topping	500 mL
¼ c.	unsweetened, shredded coconut	60 mL
¼ c.	chopped pecans	60 mL

Drain cherries, reserving liquid. Soften gelatin in the cold water. Add water to the reserved cherry liquid to make 1 c. (250 mL). Pour into a saucepan. Add softened gelatin, and stir to dissolve gelatin. Bring to a boil. Remove from heat and cool to a thick syrup. Beat until fluffy. Fold nondairy whipped topping into cherry gelatin. Fold in the cherries, coconut, and pecans. Transfer to baked pie shell. Chill for several hours or until set.

Yield: 8 servings
Exchange, 1 serving: 1⅓ bread, 2½ fat
Calories, 1 serving: 226
Carbohydrates, 1 serving: 19 g

Raspberry Cheese Pie

9 in.	baked pie shell	23 cm
1 pkg. (4-serving)	sugar-free raspberry-flavored gelatin mix	1 pkg. (4-serving)
1 T.	granulated fructose	15 mL
1¼ c.	hot water	310 mL
1-lb. bag	unsweetened, frozen raspberries	457-g bag
3 oz.	light cream cheese	85 g
2 T.	skim milk	30 mL

Dissolve gelatin and fructose in hot water. Add the frozen raspberries, and stir until berries are separated and mixture begins to thicken. Blend cream cheese with the milk. Spread cheese mixture over the bottom of the baked pie shell. Pour slightly thickened gelatin mixture over cheese. Chill until set.

Yield: 8 servings
Exchange, 1 serving: 1 bread, ½ fat, ¼ fruit
Calories, 1 serving: 138
Carbohydrates, 1 serving: 19 g

Meringue Tart-Lemon Pie

1 recipe	Meringue Pie Shell (page 88)	1 recipe
1 c.	skim milk	250 mL
½ c.	lemon juice	125 mL
1 T.	cornstarch	15 mL
½ t.	vanilla extract	2 mL
dash	salt	dash
3	egg yolks, slightly beaten	3
¾ c.	granulated sugar replacement	190 mL
	or	
½ c.	granulated fructose	125 mL
	or	
⅛ t.	Stevia Rebaudiana extract	½ mL
1 T.	grated lemon peel	15 mL

Combine milk, lemon juice, cornstarch, vanilla, and salt in a saucepan. (Mixture will appear curdled.) Cook and stir over medium heat until mixture is consistency of heavy cream. Pour a small amount of hot mixture into beaten egg yolks. Stir slightly; then pour egg yolks into hot mixture. Return to heat and cook until mixture is thick. Stir in sweetener of your choice and grated lemon peel. Remove from heat and cover. Cool completely. Pour into prepared pie shell. Chill until serving time.

Yield: 8 servings, with granulated sugar replacement or Stevia
  Rebaudiana
Exchange, 1 serving: 1/3 low-fat milk
Calories, 1 serving: 40
Carbohydrates, 1 serving: 4 g

Yield: 8 servings, with granulated fructose
Exchange, 1 serving: 1/3 low-fat milk, 2/3 fruit
Calories, 1 serving: 87
Carbohydrates, 1 serving: 14 g

Ginger Banana Pie

9 in.	baked pie shell	23 cm
6	gingersnaps	6
1 env.	unflavored gelatin	1 env.
2/3 c.	granulated sugar replacement	180 mL
3/4 c.	water	190 mL
3	bananas	3
3 T.	fresh lemon juice	45 mL
1 t.	grated lemon peel	5 mL
2	egg whites	2
	lemon juice	

Powder gingersnaps in a food processor or blender. Set aside. Combine gelatin, sugar replacement, and water in a small saucepan or microwave-safe bowl. Stir to mix. Heat until gelatin is completely dissolved. Remove from heat. Meanwhile, mash two of the bananas. Stir the 3 T. (45 mL) of lemon juice and the lemon peel into the mashed bananas. Stir banana mixture into gelatin; then allow to cool until mixture is the consistency of thick cream. Add egg whites. Beat with a rotary beater until mixture begins to hold its shape. Chill if necessary. Spoon mixture into the baked pie shell. Chill thoroughly . At serving time, slice remaining banana and dip each slice in lemon juice. Garnish top of pie with banana slices; then sprinkle with powdered gingersnaps.

Yield: 8 servings
Exchange, 1 serving: 1 bread, 1/2 fat, 2/3 fruit
Calories, 1 serving: 159
Carbohydrates, 1 serving: 23 g

Orange-Juice Angel Pie

1 recipe	Meringue Pie Shell (page 88)	1 recipe
4	egg yolks	4
1	egg	1
½ c.	granulated sugar replacement	125 mL
	or	
2 T.	granulated fructose	30 mL
¼ c.	frozen orange-juice concentrate, undiluted	60 mL
1 T.	fresh lemon juice	15 mL
2 c.	prepared nondairy whipped topping	500 mL

Beat egg yolks and egg until thick and lemon-colored. Beat in sweetener of your choice, orange-juice concentrate, and lemon juice. Pour into a saucepan. Cook and stir until mixture is very thick. Chill thoroughly. Stir slightly to loosen mixture. Fold nondairy whipped topping into cold orange mixture. Transfer to pie shell. Chill thoroughly.

Yield: 8 servings, with granulated sugar replacement
Exchange, 1 serving: ⅓ fruit, 1½ fat
Calories, 1 serving: 94
Carbohydrates, 1 serving: 4 g

Yield: 8 servings, with granulated fructose
Exchange, 1 serving: ½ fruit, 1½ fat
Calories, 1 serving: 102
Carbohydrates, 1 serving: 7 g

Buttermilk Raisin Crustless Pie

1 env.	unflavored gelatin	1 env.
¼ c.	cold water	60 mL
2 c.	buttermilk	500 mL
1 c.	raisins	250 mL
3 T.	all-purpose flour	45 mL
¼ c.	sugar-free maple-flavored syrup	60 mL
½ t.	ground cinnamon	2 mL
¼ t.	ground nutmeg	1 mL

Lightly grease the bottom and sides of a 9-in. (23-cm) pie pan. Sprinkle unflavored gelatin over cold water. Stir slightly; then allow to soften for 1 minute. Meanwhile, combine buttermilk, raisins, and flour in a saucepan. Whisk until flour is completely blended and mixture is smooth. Cook over medium-low heat until mixture is warm. Pour in softened gelatin, and continue cooking until gelatin is completely dissolved. Remove from heat. Cover and allow to cool for at least ½ hour to plump the raisins. Add maple syrup, cinnamon, and nutmeg. Pour into prepared pie pan. Bake at 350 °F (175 °C) for 45 minutes. Cool to room temperature; then chill.

Yield: 8 servings
Exchange, 1 serving: 1 fruit, ¼ low-fat milk
Calories, 1 serving: 77
Carbohydrates, 1 serving: 18 g

Blueberries-in-Milk Crustless Pie

2 c.	unsweetened, frozen blueberries	500 mL
3 T.	granulated fructose	45 mL
¾ c.	buttermilk	190 mL
¼ c.	low-fat milk	60 mL
3 T.	all-purpose flour	45 mL

Lightly grease the bottom and sides of a 9-in. (23-cm) pie pan. Place blueberries in pie pan and level. Sprinkle 1 T. (15 mL) of the granulated fructose over the top of the blueberries. Bake at 375 °F (190 °C) for 15 minutes. Meanwhile, combine remaining fructose, buttermilk, milk, and flour in a bowl. Beat or whisk until flour is completely blended and mixture is smooth. Pour buttermilk mixture over blueberries. Return to oven and continue baking for 30 minutes more or until middle of pie is just set. Cool to room temperature; then chill.

Yield: 8 servings
Exchange, 1 serving: ½ fruit, ¼ low-fat milk
Calories, 1 serving: 53
Carbohydrates, 1 serving: 10 g

Fruit Desserts

Fruit Platter with Mango Sauce

2 large	mangos, pitted	2 large
⅓ c.	unsweetened pineapple juice	90 mL
2 T.	fresh lime juice	30 mL
1 T.	granulated fructose	15 mL
2	papayas (peeled, seeded, and cut into 12 slices)	2
1	pineapple (peeled, cored, and cut into 12 slices)	1
1	honeydew melon (peeled and cut into 12 wedges)	1
1 T.	grated lime peel	30 mL

Cut away mango flesh from skin. Combine mango, pineapple juice, lime juice, and fructose in a blender. Process to a puree. Cover and refrigerate. Arrange papaya slices, pineapple slices, and honeydew wedges on a large platter. Pour mango sauce over fruit. Sprinkle with lime peel.

Yield: 12 servings
Exchange, 1 serving: 2 fruit
Calories, 1 serving: 126
Carbohydrates, 1 serving: 26 g

Fruit Chutney

1 c.	raspberry vinegar	250 mL
½ c.	red-wine vinegar	125 mL
2 c.	dry white wine	500 mL
½ c.	frozen orange-juice concentrate	125 mL

1 c.	crushed pineapple in juice	250 mL
1 c.	diced apple	250 mL
⅔ c.	diced papaya	180 mL
⅔ c.	diced mango	180 mL
½ c.	thinly sliced green bell pepper	125 mL
½ c.	thinly sliced red bell pepper	125 mL
½ c.	thinly sliced yellow bell pepper	125 mL
¼ c.	granulated sugar replacement	60 mL
6 whole	peppercorns	6 whole
1	bay leaf	1
2 T.	minced fresh mint	30 mL

Combine vinegars in a large saucepan. Bring to a boil, reduce heat, and simmer to reduce liquid to about ½ c. (125 mL). Add wine, orange-juice concentrate, fruit, bell peppers, sugar replacement, peppercorns, and bay leaf. Cook until fruit is soft. Transfer fruit and bell peppers to a bowl. Simmer liquid for about 5 minutes. Return fruit and bell peppers to saucepan. Cook over low heat, stirring occasionally, and reduce mixture to about 2½ c. Remove from heat. Remove peppercorns and bay leaf. Stir in mint. Cover and chill.

Yield: 20 servings
Exchange, 1 serving: negligible
Calories, 1 serving: negligible
Carbohydrates, 1 serving: negligible

Glazed Apricots

½ c.	water	125 mL
2 T.	all-natural orange marmalade	30 mL
16	moist dried apricots	16

Combine water and marmalade in a small nonstick saucepan. Heat and stir over medium heat until marmalade is melted. Add apricots. Reduce heat; then cover and simmer until apricots are tender and syrup is reduced and coats apricots (about 20 to 25 minutes). Cool apricots in syrup. Remove apricots from syrup. Drain to remove excess syrup.

Yield: 8 servings
Exchange, 1 serving: ½ fruit
Calories, 1 serving: 24
Carbohydrates, 1 serving: 6 g

Cranberry and Raspberry Fool

1½ c.	fresh cranberries	375 mL
1½ c.	fresh raspberries	375 mL
¼ c.	granulated fructose	60 mL
¼ c.	raspberry juice	60 mL
2 c.	prepared nondairy whipped topping	500 mL

Combine cranberries, raspberries, and fructose in a food processor or blender. Process into a puree. Transfer to a nonstick saucepan. Stir in raspberry juice. Cook and stir over medium heat until mixture is a thick puree. If desired, press through a sieve to remove seeds. Transfer mixture to a large bowl. Cover and chill mixture thoroughly. To serve: Swirl nondairy whipped topping into cranberry-raspberry mixture. Do not mix thoroughly. Divide evenly among six decorative glasses. Serve immediately.

Yield: 6 servings
Exchange, 1 serving: ⅓ fruit, 1 fat
Calories, 1 serving: 69
Carbohydrates, 1 serving: 4 g

Poached Bananas in Apple Juice

2 c.	apple juice	500 mL
2 T.	raisins	30 mL
1 T.	vanilla extract	15 mL
1 stick	cinnamon	1 stick
4	firm ripe bananas, cut in half	4
8 T.	nonfat plain yogurt	120 mL

Combine apple juice, raisins, vanilla, and cinnamon in a saucepan. Bring to a light boil. Reduce heat and simmer for 5 minutes. Add bananas; then cover and simmer 6 to 8 minutes or until bananas are just tender. Spoon each half-banana into a small dessert bowl or plate. Remove cinnamon stick from sauce. Divide sauce evenly among the plates. Top each plate with 1 T. (15 mL) of yogurt. Serve immediately.

Yield: 8 servings
Exchange, 1 serving: 1¼ fruit
Calories, 1 serving: 75
Carbohydrates, 1 serving: 18 g

Strawberries with Cinnamon Sauce

⅔ c.	water	180 mL
1 t.	ground cinnamon	5 mL
6 in.	cinnamon stick, broken in pieces	9 cm
1 T.	cold water	15 mL
1 t.	cornstarch	5 mL
3 env.	aspartame sweetener	3 env.
2 c.	frozen, unsweetened strawberries*	500 mL
2 T.	prepared nondairy whipped topping	30 mL

*This recipe can be made with fresh strawberries, but there will be less juice.

Combine the ⅔ c. (180 mL) of water and the ground cinnamon and broken cinnamon pieces in a saucepan. Bring to a boil, reduce heat, and simmer until liquid is about ½ c. (125 mL). Remove cinnamon pieces. Dissolve the cornstarch in the 1 T. (15 mL) of cold water. Pour into cinnamon water. Cook and stir until mixture becomes the consistency of a thin syrup. Remove from heat. Allow to cool until pan is cool enough to comfortably put on your hand. Stir in the aspartame sweetener. Place frozen strawberries in a narrow bowl. Pour warm cinnamon mixture over the strawberries. Cover and refrigerate until strawberries are thawed and liquid is chilled. To serve: Divide berries and juice evenly between two decorative glasses. Top each glass with 1 T. (15 mL) of nondairy whipped topping.

Yield: 2 servings
Exchange, 1 serving: 1 fruit
Calories, 1 serving: 55
Carbohydrates, 1 serving: 13 g

Puddings

Easy German Rice Pudding

½ c.	long-grain rice	125 mL
1 c.	boiling water	250 mL
3 c.	skim milk	750 mL
½ c.	granulated sugar replacement	125 mL
	or	
1 T.	liquid Stevia Rebaudiana extract (page 8)	15 mL
½ t.	salt	2 mL
1 t.	vanilla extract	5 mL
	ground cinnamon	

Combine rice and boiling water in a 2-qt. (2-L) saucepan. Bring to a boil; then reduce heat and cook, uncovered, until all the water is absorbed. Stir occasionally. Stir in the milk. Simmer for 20 minutes, stirring occasionally. Add sweetener of your choice and salt. Continue simmering 20 to 25 more minutes or until mixture is creamy and very soft. Stir in vanilla. Serve warm, sprinkled with ground cinnamon.

Yield: 4 servings
Exchange, 1 serving: 1 bread, ¾ skim milk
Calories, 1 serving: 150
Carbohydrates, 1 serving: 29 g

Baked Apple Pudding

1 c.	granulated sugar replacement	250 mL
	or	
⅛ t.	Stevia Rebaudiana extract	½ mL
2	eggs	2

98

1 T.	liquid fructose	15 mL
2 t.	vanilla extract	10 mL
⅓ c.	all-purpose flour	90 mL
1 T.	baking powder	15 mL
dash	salt	dash
3 c.	chopped pared apples	750 mL

Combine sweetener of your choice, eggs, liquid fructose, and vanilla in a bowl. Beat until thick. Stir in flour, baking powder, and salt. Then stir in apples. Spread batter into a well-greased 9-in. (23-cm)-square baking pan. Bake at 325 °F (165 °C) for 25 to 35 minutes or until done. Serve warm.

Yield: 12 servings
Exchange, 1 serving: 1 fruit
Calories, 1 serving: 52
Carbohydrates, 1 serving: 12 g

Milk-Chocolate Pudding

1 c.	granulated sugar replacement	250 mL
	or	
⅛ t.	Stevia Rebaudiana extract	½ mL
⅔ c.	all-purpose flour	180 mL
¼ c.	unsweetened baking cocoa	60 mL
2 T.	liquid fructose	30 mL
dash	salt	dash
1 qt.	skim milk	1 L
1	egg, beaten	1
1 T.	vanilla extract	15 mL

Combine sweetener of your choice, flour, cocoa, fructose, and salt in a nonstick saucepan. Combine milk and egg in measuring cup or bowl. Stir to blend. Gradually stir milk mixture into cocoa mixture. Cook over medium heat until mixture thickens, stirring constantly. Remove from heat, and stir in vanilla. Spoon into eight decorative dessert dishes. Serve warm or chill until set.

Yield: 8 servings
Exchange, 1 serving: ½ bread, ½ low-fat milk
Calories, 1 serving: 117
Carbohydrates, 1 serving: 13 g

Caramel Custard

1 T.	sugar-free maple-flavored syrup	15 mL
1	egg	1
½ c.	evaporated skim milk	125 mL
⅓ c.	water	90 mL
1 T.	granulated sugar replacement	15 mL
1 t.	vanilla extract	5 mL
dash	salt	dash

Divide maple syrup evenly between two custard cups. Combine egg, milk, water, sugar replacement, vanilla, and salt in a mixing bowl. Beat to blend. Carefully pour custard mixture over the syrup in the custard cups. Set cups in shallow pan holding 1 in. (2.5 cm) of water. Bake at 350 °F (175 °C) for 50 minutes or until knife inserted in middle comes out clean.

Microwave: Water bath not needed. Prepare recipe as above. Place custard cups on a flat microwave-proof plate. Cook on LOW for 8 to 10 minutes or until edges are set and middle is soft but not runny. Allow to cool for 10 to 15 minutes before serving.

Yield: 2 servings
Exchange, 1 serving: 1 skim milk
Calories, 1 serving: 85
Carbohydrates, 1 serving: 7 g

Baked Coffee Custard

1¼ c.	low fat milk	310 mL
¼ c.	liquid nondairy creamer	60 mL
4 t.	instant coffee powder	20 mL
2	eggs	2
2	egg yolks	2
2 T.	granulated sugar replacement	30 mL
1 T.	granulated fructose	15 mL
dash	salt	dash
1 T.	vanilla extract	15 mL

Place six custard cups in a large baking pan. Place pan with custard cups in a 325 °F (165 °C) oven. Meanwhile, heat the milk and nondairy creamer until boiling. Remove from heat and stir in the coffee powder. Set aside. Whisk the eggs and egg yolks together in a bowl. Add sugar replacement, fructose, salt, and vanilla. Whisk to thoroughly blend. Gradually whisk in the hot milk. Remove baking pan and custard cups from oven. Divide the coffee mixture evenly among the custard cups. Pour simmering water into baking pan to come halfway up sides of custard cups. Return to oven. Bake for 35 minutes or until the middle moves only slightly. Remove custard cups from baking pan. Cool.

Yield: 6 servings
Exchange, 1 serving: ½ low-fat milk, 1 fat
Calories, 1 serving: 113
Carbohydrates, 1 serving: 7 g

Mocha Mousse

⅓ c.	unsweetened cocoa powder	90 mL
1 t.	instant-coffee powder	5 mL
¼ c.	granulated sugar replacement	60 mL
2 T.	cornstarch	30 mL
¼ t.	salt	1 mL
2 c.	skim milk	500 mL
1	beaten egg	1
8-oz. pkg.	light cream cheese, softened	240-g pkg.
1 t.	vanilla extract	5 mL

Combine cocoa powder, coffee powder, sugar replacement, cornstarch, and salt in a saucepan. Stir in milk. Cook and stir over medium heat until thick and bubbling. Reduce heat to low. Cook and stir 4 minutes more. Remove from heat. Pour and stir a small amount of hot cocoa mixture into the beaten egg. Pour egg mixture back into cocoa mixture, stirring until well blended. Return to heat and cook for 2 more minutes. Remove from heat. Pour mixture into a mixing bowl. Add cream cheese and vanilla. Beat until fluffy and mixture is well blended. Pour into a 1-qt. (1-L) mould or dish, and cover with waxed paper. Chill until firm. Remove waxed paper and unmould.

Yield: 10 servings
Exchange, 1 serving: 1 whole milk, 1 fat
Calories, 1 serving: 128
Carbohydrates, 1 serving: 13 g

Dark-Fudge Pudding

½ c.	granulated sugar replacement	125 mL
3 T.	all-purpose flour	45 mL
1 T.	granulated fructose	15 mL
dash	salt	dash
1½ c.	skim milk	375 mL
1 oz.	unsweetened baking chocolate, in small pieces	28.3 g
1	egg, beaten	1
1 T.	margarine	15 mL
1 t.	vanilla extract	5 mL

Combine sugar replacement, flour, fructose, and salt in a nonstick sauce-pan. Gradually stir in milk. Blend well. Stir in chocolate and egg. Cook over medium heat until mixture thickens, stirring constantly. Remove from heat, and stir in margarine and vanilla. Spoon into six decorative dessert dishes. Serve warm or chill until set.

Yield: 6 servings
Exchange, 1 serving: 1 bread, ½ fat
Calories, 1 serving: 108
Carbohydrates, 1 serving: 14 g

Fluffy Rice Pudding

½ c.	water	125 mL
½ c.	granulated sugar replacement	125 mL
2 T.	granulated fructose	30 mL
2 env.	unflavored gelatin	2 env.
½ t.	salt	2 mL
2 c.	skim milk	500 mL
1½ c.	cooked rice	375 mL
1 T.	vanilla extract	15 mL
2 c.	prepared nondairy whipped topping	500 mL

Combine water, sugar replacement, fructose, gelatin, and salt in a sauce-pan. Heat, stirring constantly until gelatin is dissolved. Stir in milk, rice, and vanilla. Place saucepan in a bowl of iced water. Stir occasionally. When rice mixture has cooled and drops in mounds from a spoon, fold in nondairy whipped topping. Pour into 6-c. (1500-mL) decorative mould.

Cover with plastic wrap and refrigerate until firm. Loosen edges of mould with a spatula, and dip mould briefly in a pan of warm water. Invert on decorative serving plate.

Yield: 12 servings
Exchange, 1 serving: 1 bread
Calories, 1 serving: 78
Carbohydrates, 1 serving: 12 g

Rhubarb Bread Pudding

1 qt.	diced rhubarb	1 L
3½ c.	dry bread cubes	875 mL
1 c.	granulated sugar replacement	250 mL
	or	
⅛ t.	Stevia Rebaudiana extract	½ mL
¼ c.	margarine, melted	60 mL
2 T.	granulated fructose	30 mL
½ t.	ground nutmeg	2 mL
½ t.	ground cinnamon	2 mL
¼ t.	ground allspice	1 mL

Combine all ingredients in a bowl. Toss to mix. Transfer to a well-greased 2-qt. (2-L) casserole dish. Cover and bake at 375 °F (190 °C) for 45 minutes, then uncover and continue baking another 10 minutes or until set. Serve warm.

Yield: 8 servings
Exchange, 1 serving: 1⅓ bread, 1 fat
Calories, 1 serving: 148
Carbohydrates, 1 serving: 21 g

Cookies

Raisin Oatmeal Cookies

1 c.	all-purpose flour	250 mL
1 t.	ground cinnamon	5 mL
½ t.	baking powder	2 mL
½ t.	baking soda	2 mL
¼ t.	salt	1 mL
½ c. (1 stick)	solid margarine, softened	125 mL (1 stick)
2 T.	granulated fructose	30 mL
1 large	egg	1 large
1 t.	vanilla extract	5 mL
1 c.	granulated sugar replacement or	250 mL
⅛ t.	Stevia Rebaudiana extract	½ mL
1¼ c.	quick-cooking oatmeal	310 mL
½ c.	raisins	125 mL

Combine flour, cinnamon, baking powder, baking soda, and salt in a bowl. Stir to mix. Combine margarine, fructose, egg, and vanilla in a mixing bowl. Beat until thoroughly blended. Beat in sweetener of your choice. Gradually add flour mixture. Beat until blended. Meanwhile, combine oatmeal and raisins in a bowl. Work with your fingers or a spoon to separate the raisins and coat them with the oatmeal. Beat into cookie mixture. Drop by tablespoonfuls onto an ungreased cookie sheet. Bake at 375 °F (190 °C) for 10 to 12 minutes. Cool slightly on cookie sheet; then move to cooling rack.

Yield: 36 cookies
Exchange, 1 cookie: ½ bread, ¼ fat
Calories, 1 cookie: 61
Carbohydrates, 1 cookie: 7 g

Carob Cookies

1¼ c.	all-purpose flour	310 mL
⅓ c.	powdered carob	90 mL
½ t.	baking soda	2 mL
¼ t.	salt	1 mL
½ c.	margarine, softened	125 mL
½ c.	granulated fructose	125 mL
1	egg	1
1 t.	vanilla extract	5 mL

Combine flour, carob, baking soda, and salt in mixing bowl. In another mixing bowl, cream margarine and fructose. Next, beat in egg and vanilla extract. Then gradually beat in flour mixture. Drop onto an ungreased cookie sheet. Bake at 350 °F (175 °C) for 10 to 12 minutes. Allow to cool on cookie sheet for 2 minutes before removing to a cooling rack.

Yield: 36 cookies
Exchange, 1 cookie: ¼ bread, ⅓ fat
Calories, 1 cookie: 45
Carbohydrates, 1 cookie: 4 g

Carob-Chip Cookies

1½ c.	all-purpose flour	375 mL
¾ t.	baking powder	4 mL
½ t.	salt	2 mL
¾ c.	margarine, softened	190 mL
½ c.	granulated fructose	125 mL
1	egg	1
1 t.	vanilla extract	5 mL
½ c.	unsweetened carob mini-chips	125 mL

Combine flour, baking powder, and salt in mixing bowl. In another mixing bowl, cream margarine and fructose; then beat in egg and vanilla extract. Gradually beat flour mixture into creamed mixture Stir in carob chips. Drop onto an ungreased cookie sheet. Bake at 375 °F (190 °C) for 8 to 10 minutes. Allow to cool on cookie sheet for 2 minutes before removing to a cooling rack.

Yield: 36 cookies
Exchange, 1 cookie: ¼ bread, ½ fat
Calories, 1 cookie: 43
Carbohydrates, 1 cookie: 4 g

Pecan Cookies

8-oz. pkg.	light cream cheese	227-g pkg.
3 T.	granulated fructose	45 mL
1 t.	vanilla extract	5 mL
1	egg	1
1	egg white	1
1 c.	all-purpose flour	250 mL
½ t.	baking soda	2 mL
½ t.	baking powder	2 mL
⅓ c.	sugar-free white frosting mix	90 mL
48	pecan halves	48
¼ c.	sugar-free white frosting mix	60 mL
1 T.	water	15 mL

Combine cream cheese, fructose, and vanilla in a mixing bowl. Beat until fluffy. Beat in egg and egg white. Beat at least 3 minutes. Combine flour, baking soda, baking powder, and the ⅓ c. (90 mL) of white frosting mix in a bowl. Stir to mix. (Break up any lumps in frosting mix.) Gradually beat flour mixture into cream-cheese mixture. Cover with plastic wrap and refrigerate at least 3 hours or until completely chilled. Drop by teaspoonfuls onto an ungreased cookie sheet. Bake at 325 °F (165 °C) for 15 to 20 minutes. Remove from pan immediately. Press one pecan half into the middle of each cookie. Combine the ¼ c. (60 mL) of white frosting mix and water in a cup. Stir to blend into a glaze. Add extra water if needed. Lightly brush a glaze on each cookie. Move to cooling rack.

Yield: 48 cookies
Exchange, 1 cookie: ⅓ bread, ¼ fat
Calories, 1 cookie: 30
Carbohydrates, 1 cookie: 4 g

Chocolate Softies

8-oz. pkg.	light cream cheese	227-g pkg.
2 oz.	semisweet baking chocolate, melted	57 g
3 T.	granulated fructose	45 mL
1 t.	vanilla extract	5 mL
1	egg	1
1	egg white	1
1¼ c.	all-purpose flour	310 mL
½ t.	baking soda	2 mL
½ t.	baking powder	2 mL

Combine cream cheese, melted baking chocolate, fructose, and vanilla in a mixing bowl. Beat until fluffy. Beat in egg and egg white. Beat at least 3 minutes. Combine flour, baking soda, and baking powder in a bowl. Stir to mix. Gradually beat flour mixture into cream-cheese mixture. Cover with plastic wrap and refrigerate at least 3 hours or until completely chilled. Drop by teaspoonfuls onto an ungreased cookie sheet. Bake at 325 °F (165 °C) for 15 to 20 minutes. Remove from pan and place on cooling rack immediately.

Yield: 48 cookies
Exchange, 1 cookie: ⅙ bread, ⅓ fat
Calories, 1 cookie: 31
Carbohydrates, 1 cookie: 2 g

Applesauce Spice Cookies

2 c.	cake flour	500 mL
1 t.	baking powder	5 mL
½ t.	baking soda	2 mL
½ t.	ground cinnamon	2 mL
¼ t.	ground cloves	1 mL
¼ t.	ground nutmeg	1 mL
¼ t.	salt	1 mL
½ c.	solid margarine	125 mL
(1 stick)		(1 stick)
2 T.	granulated fructose	30 mL
1 large	egg	1 large
¾ c.	granulated sugar replacement	190 mL
	or	
⅛ t.	Stevia Rebaudiana extract	½ mL
1 c.	unsweetened applesauce	250 mL

Sift cake flour, baking powder, baking soda, cinnamon, cloves, nutmeg, and salt into a bowl. Combine margarine and fructose in a mixing bowl. Beat until creamy. Beat in egg and sweetener of your choice. Add flour mixture alternately with applesauce to creamed mixture, beginning and ending with flour mixture. Drop on a well-greased cookie sheet. Bake at 375 °F (190 °C) for 12 to 15 minutes.

Yield: 36 cookies
Exchange, 1 cookie: ⅓ bread, ½ fat
Calories, 1 cookie: 57
Carbohydrates, 1 cookie: 4 g

Chocolate Thins

¼ c.	solid margarine, softened	60 mL
4 t.	granulated sugar replacement	20 mL
1	egg	1
2 T.	unsweetened cocoa powder	30 mL
1 t.	vanilla extract	5 mL
1 c.	all-purpose flour	250 mL
1 t.	baking powder	5 mL
¼ t.	baking soda	1 mL
dash	salt	dash
2 T.	water	30 mL

Combine margarine, sugar replacement, egg, cocoa, and vanilla in a mixing bowl or food processor. With an electric mixer or steel blade, process until creamy. Add flour, baking powder, baking soda, salt, and water. Mix well. Shape dough into two balls. Wrap each ball in plastic wrap and refrigerate at least 2 hours or overnight. Roll out dough to ⅛-in. (3-mm) thickness on a lightly floured surface. Cut with a 2½-in. (6.25-cm) round cookie cutter and place on ungreased cookie sheets. Bake at 350 °F (175 °C) for 8 to 10 minutes.

Yield: 30 cookies
Exchange, 1 cookie: ⅕ bread, ⅕ fat
Calories, 1 cookie: 22
Carbohydrates, 1 cookie: 2 g

Hazelnut Cookies

8-oz. pkg.	light cream cheese	227-g pkg.
3 T.	granulated fructose	45 mL
1 t.	vanilla extract	5 mL
1	egg	1
1	egg white	1
1 c.	all-purpose flour	250 mL
½ t.	baking soda	2 mL
½ t.	baking powder	2 mL
⅓ c.	finely ground hazelnuts	90 mL

Combine cream cheese, fructose, and vanilla in a mixing bowl. Beat until fluffy. Beat in egg and egg white. Beat at least 3 minutes. Combine flour, baking soda, and baking powder in a bowl. Stir to mix. Gradually beat flour mixture into cream-cheese mixture. Stir in ground hazelnuts. Cover with plastic wrap and refrigerate at least 3 hours or until completely chilled. Drop by teaspoonfuls onto an ungreased cookie sheet. Bake at 325 °F (165 °C) for 15 to 20 minutes. Remove from pan and place on cooling rack immediately.

Yield: 48 cookies
Exchange, 1 cookie: ⅙ bread, ½ fat
Calories, 1 cookie: 34
Carbohydrates, 1 cookie: 2 g

Sweet "Sugar" Cookies

2 c.	all-purpose flour	500 mL
½ t.	baking powder	2 mL
½ t.	baking soda	2 mL
¼ t.	salt	1 mL
½ c.	solid vegetable shortening	125 mL
¾ c.	granulated sugar replacement	190 mL
	or	
⅛ t.	Stevia Rebaudiana extract	½ mL
1 large	egg	1 large
3 T.	skim milk	15 mL
1 t.	vanilla extract	5 mL
1 t.	grated orange peel	5 mL
3 env.	aspartame sweetener	3 env.

Sift the flour, baking powder, baking soda, and salt together into a bowl. Combine the solid shortening and sweetener of your choice in a mixing bowl. Beat until creamy. Beat in the egg, milk, vanilla extract, and orange peel. Blend in the flour mixture. Lightly grease two large cookie sheets. Roll dough out on a lightly floured surface to ⅛-in. (8-mm) thickness. Cut with a doughnut cutter. Transfer dough rounds to prepared cookie sheets. Gather and reroll scraps. Cut additional cookies. Bake at 375 °F (190 °C) for 14 minutes or until edges of cookies are golden brown. Remove from oven. Sprinkle cookies with aspartame sweetener (use one envelope for eight cookies). Move cookies to cooling rack. For a festive holiday touch, sprinkle cookies with a small amount of colored sugar-free gelatin.

Yield: 24 cookies
Exchange, 1 cookie: ½ bread, ¼ fat
Calories, 1 cookie: 46
Carbohydrates, 1 cookie: 7 g

Vanilla Wafers

¼ c.	solid margarine, softened	60 mL
4 t.	granulated sugar replacement	20 mL
1	egg	1
1 T.	vanilla extract	15 mL
1 c.	all-purpose flour	250 mL
1 t.	baking powder	5 mL
¼ t.	baking soda	1 mL
dash	salt	dash
2 T.	water	30 mL

Combine margarine, sugar replacement, egg, and vanilla in a mixing bowl or food processor. With an electric mixer or steel blade, process until creamy. Add flour, baking powder, baking soda, salt, and water. Mix well. Shape dough into two balls. Wrap each ball in plastic wrap and refrigerate at least 2 hours or overnight. Roll out dough to ⅛-in. (3-mm) thickness on a lightly floured surface. Cut with a 2½-in. (6.25-cm) round cookie cutter and place on ungreased cookie sheets. Bake at 350 °F (175 °C) for 8 to 10 minutes.

Yield: 30 cookies
Exchange, 1 cookie: ⅕ bread, ⅕ fat
Calories, 1 cookie: 21
Carbohydrates, 1 cookie: 2 g

Lemon-Sandwich Cookies

Cookie:

½ c.	solid margarine	125 mL
½ c.	granulated sugar replacement	125 mL
	or	
1 T.	liquid Stevia Rebaudiana extract (page 8)	15 mL
2	eggs	2
1 T.	lemon juice	15 mL
1 t.	vanilla extract	5 mL
1½ c.	all-purpose flour	375 mL
¼ t.	baking soda	1 mL
dash	salt	dash

Combine margarine, sweetener of your choice, eggs, lemon juice, and vanilla in a mixing bowl. Beat to blend. Stir in flour, baking soda, and salt. Work into a soft, smooth dough. Divide dough in half. Shape each half into a 7 × 1½ in. (17.5 × 3.75 cm) roll. Wrap in plastic wrap and chill for 8 hours or overnight. Cut each roll into approximately ⅛-in. (3-mm) slices, or cut 48 slices from each roll. Place on ungreased cookie sheet. Bake at 400 °F (200 °C) for 5 to 6 minutes or until edges begin to brown. Cool completely before filling.

Filling:

⅓ c.	sugar-free white frosting-mix powder	90 mL
1 t.	grated lemon peel	5 mL
1 T.	hot lemon juice	15 mL
	yellow food coloring	

Combine frosting-mix powder, lemon peel, hot lemon juice, and yellow food coloring in a small bowl. Beat with a small wire whisk or fork until smooth. Put cookies together in pairs with filling.

Yield: 48 cookies
Exchange, 1 cookie: ⅓ bread, ⅓ fat
Calories, 1 cookie: 41
Carbohydrates, 1 cookie: 4 g

Fancies

3	eggs	3
1 c.	granulated sugar replacement	250 mL
3 T.	granulated fructose	45 mL
½ t.	salt	2 mL
3 T.	melted shortening	45 mL
1 T.	vanilla extract	15 mL
3 c.	quick-cooking oatmeal	750 mL

Beat eggs until lemon-colored. Gradually beat in sugar replacement and fructose. Beat in salt, melted shortening, and vanilla. Beat well. Beat in oatmeal. Drop teaspoonfuls onto a greased cookie sheet. Bake at 325 °F (165 °C) for 17 to 20 minutes or until done. Move from pan to cooling rack while still warm.

Yield: 110 tea cookies
Exchange, 1 cookie: ⅙ bread
Calories, 1 cookie: 13
Carbohydrates, 1 cookie: 2 g

Crisscross Peanut-Butter Cookies

1½ c.	all-purpose flour	375 mL
½ t.	baking powder	2 mL
1 c.	low-sugar creamy peanut butter	250 mL
½ c.	solid margarine	125 mL
(1 stick)		(1 stick)
2 T.	granulated fructose	30 mL
1 large	egg	1 large
1 t.	vanilla extract	5 mL
1 c.	granulated sugar replacement	250 mL
	or	
⅛ t.	Stevia Rebaudiana extract	½ mL

Combine flour and baking powder in a bowl. Stir to mix. Combine peanut butter, margarine, and fructose in a mixing bowl. Beat until creamy. Beat in egg, vanilla, and sweetener of your choice. Gradually add the flour mixture. (If you are using a hand mixer, you may have to stir the last part of the flour into the cookie dough.) Roll teaspoons of dough into a ball. Place on ungreased cookie sheets. Flatten with a fork in a crisscross design. Bake at 375 °F (190 °C) for 10 to 12 minutes or until cookies are golden brown. Cool slightly on cookie sheet. Then move to cooling rack.

Yield: 60 cookies
Exchange, 1 cookie: ⅕ bread, 1 fat
Calories, 1 cookie: 62
Carbohydrates, 1 cookie: 2 g

Butter-Nut Drops

½ c.	solid margarine	125 mL
2 T.	granulated fructose	30 mL
1	egg, separated	1
½ t.	vanilla extract	2 mL
¼ t.	salt	1 mL
1 c.	cake flour	250 mL
1 T.	lemon juice	15 mL
2 T.	grated orange peel	30 mL
1 T.	grated lemon peel	15 mL
½ c.	Brazil nuts, finely ground	125 mL

Cream margarine and fructose together. Beat in egg yolk and vanilla. Beat in salt, cake flour, and lemon juice. Add grated orange and lemon peels.

Form into a ball and wrap in plastic wrap. Chill thoroughly (at least 2 to 3 hours). Roll dough into tiny balls (about ½ t. [2 mL] of dough per ball). Dip each ball into the slightly beaten egg white. Roll in the ground nuts. Place on lightly greased cookie sheets about 1 in. (2.5 cm) apart. Press top slightly with your finger. Bake at 350 °F (175 °C) for 20 to 25 minutes.

Yield: 25 cookies
Exchange, 1 cookie: ⅓ bread, ½ fat
Calories, 1 cookie: 50
Carbohydrates, 1 cookie: 2 g

Date Crumb Bars

8-oz. pkg.	chopped dates	227-g pkg.
⅔ c.	water	180 mL
2 t.	vanilla extract	10 mL
1½ c.	all-purpose flour	375 mL
1½ c.	quick-cooking oatmeal	375 mL
¾ c.	granulated sugar replacement	190 mL
¾ t.	baking soda	4 mL
¼ t.	salt	1 mL
¾ c.	solid margarine	190 mL

Combine dates and water in a saucepan. Bring to a boil, reduce heat, and simmer until mixture is thick and dates are very soft. Remove from heat and stir in the vanilla. Cool. Combine flour, oatmeal, sugar replacement, baking soda, and salt in a mixing bowl. Add margarine and work with your fingers or a spoon until mixture becomes coarse crumbs. Transfer about two-thirds of the crumb mixture to a greased 9 × 13 in. (23 × 33 cm) baking pan. Reserve remaining crumbs. Firmly press crumb mixture on bottom of pan. Spoon date mixture in large dots around pressed-crumb surface. Using the back of a dampened wooden spoon or a dampened pastry brush, spread date filling over crumb crust. (Occasionally redampening spoon or brush will aid in spreading the filling over the entire surface.) Sprinkle the remaining crumbs over the date filling. Press crumbs lightly into filling. Bake at 350 °F (175 °C) for 25 to 25 minutes or until top is golden brown. Cool in pan.

Yield: 36 bars
Exchange, 1 bar: ½ bread, ¾ fat
Calories, 1 bar: 78
Carbohydrates, 1 bar: 7 g

Fudgy Bars

1½ c.	all-purpose flour	375 mL
2 t.	baking powder	10 mL
½ t.	salt	2 mL
1 c.	solid margarine	250 mL
(2 sticks)		(2 sticks)
4 oz.	unsweetened baking chocolate	113 g
¼ t.	Stevia Rebaudiana extract powder	1 mL
1½ T.	granulated fructose	21 mL
3 large	eggs	3 large
2	egg whites	2
2 t.	vanilla extract	10 mL

Combine flour, baking powder, and salt in a bowl, and mix slightly. Set aside. Combine margarine and baking chocolate either in a large microwave-safe bowl or a saucepan. Heat until chocolate is melted. Stir until smooth. Beat in Stevia Rebaudiana and fructose. Combine eggs and egg whites in a smaller bowl. Beat with a fork or wire whisk until blended. Gradually pour eggs into chocolate mixture, beating after each addition. Add vanilla. Beat in the flour mixture. Continue beating until smooth. Transfer to a greased 9 × 13 in. (23 × 33 cm) baking pan. Bake at 350 °F (175 °C) for 20 to 25 minutes or until toothpick inserted in middle comes out with moist crumbs. Cool in pan.

Optional: 1-c. (250-mL) chopped walnuts. Stir walnuts into batter before baking.

Optional: 4.5-oz. (128-g) package of sugar-free chocolate frosting mix. Prepare as directed on package. Frost after bars have cooled.

Yield: 36 bars
Exchange, 1 bar: ¼ bread, ½ fat
Calories, 1 bar: 47
Carbohydrates, 1 bar: 4 g

Yield: 36 bars, with walnuts
Exchange, 1 bar: ¼ bread, 1 fat
Calories, 1 bar: 66
Carbohydrates, 1 bar: 4 g

Yield: 36 bars, with chocolate frosting
Exchange, 1 bar: ½ bread, ½ fat
Calories, 1 bar: 61
Carbohydrates, 1 bar: 7 g

Bells for Christmas

¼ c.	solid margarine	60 mL
(½ stick)		(½ stick)
¼ c.	solid vegetable shortening	60 mL
½ c.	granulated sugar replacement	125 mL
	or	
1 T.	liquid Stevia Rebaudiana extract (page 8)	15 mL
1	egg	1
1 t.	vanilla extract	5 mL
1½ c.	all-purpose flour	375 mL
¼ t.	baking soda	1 mL
dash	salt	dash
	red or green food coloring	

Combine margarine, shortening, sweetener of your choice, egg, and vanilla in a mixing bowl. Beat to blend. Stir in flour, baking soda, and salt. Transfer about two-thirds of the dough to another bowl, and color with several drops of food coloring. (The dough will be stiff. Work dough with a spoon or fork; then knead dough to incorporate the coloring completely.) Shape colored dough into a 10 × 1½ in. (25 × 3.75 cm) roll. Knead remaining uncolored dough until soft. Roll out on a lightly floured surface into a 11 × 6 in. (27.5 × 15 cm) rectangle. Lightly brush surface with water. Wrap uncolored dough around the colored dough roll. Do not wrap the ends of the roll. Cut away any excess dough from seam edge and side edges. Reserve cut-away dough. Dampen edge of dough along 10-in. (25-cm) side of roll. Press edges of dough together to tighten. Carefully roll entire cookie roll to secure the doughs together. Wrap in plastic wrap. With the handle of a wooden spoon or your hands, carefully form the dough into a bell by pressing the top of the roll together slightly and leaving the lower half flared and curved like the bottom of a bell. Refrigerate at least 8 hours or overnight. Cut roll into about ⅛-in. (3-mm) slices. Place cookies on ungreased cookie sheets. Form a very small amount of the reserved dough into a ball to make the clapper for the bell. Place clapper on the bottom edge of bell. Bake at 375 °F (190 °C) for 7 to 8 minutes or until edges are lightly browned. Move cookies to cooling rack.

Yield: 60 cookies
Exchange, 1 cookie: ⅙ bread, ½ fat
Calories, 1 cookie: 29
Carbohydrates, 1 cookie: 2 g

Candy

Coconut Candy

1¼ c.	unsweetened coconut, grated	310 mL
½ c.	milk	125 mL
2 t.	unflavored gelatin	10 mL
1 t.	cornstarch	5 mL
1 t.	white vanilla extract	5 mL
1 recipe	Semisweet Dipping Chocolate (opposite page)	1 recipe

Combine ¼ c. (60 mL) of the coconut and the milk, gelatin, and cornstarch in a blender, and blend until smooth. Pour into small saucepan; cook and stir over medium heat until slightly thickened. Remove from heat and stir in vanilla and remaining coconut. Form into 16 patties, and allow to cool completely. Dip into chocolate.

Yield: 16 candies
Exchange, 1 candy: ⅓ whole milk, ½ fat
Calories, 1 candy: 66
Carbohydrates, 1 candy: 4 g

Crunch Candy

6 large	shredded-wheat biscuits	6 large
1 t.	unflavored gelatin	5 mL
¾ c.	cold milk	190 mL
½ c.	creamy peanut butter	125 mL
1 recipe	Semisweet Dipping Chocolate (opposite page)	1 recipe

Break shredded-wheat biscuits into small pieces. Set aside. Soak gelatin in ¼ c. (60 mL) of the cold milk; set aside. Combine peanut butter and remaining milk in top of a double boiler and place over hot (not boiling) water. Cook and stir until smooth. Add soaked gelatin; then cook and stir until gelatin is completely dissolved and smooth. Fold reserved shredded-wheat pieces into peanut-butter mixture. Drop by teaspoonfuls onto lightly greased waxed paper. Allow to firm and cool; then dip in chocolate.

Yield: 32 candies
Exchange, 1 candy: ⅓ whole milk
Calories, 1 candy: 44
Carbohydrates, 1 candy: 4 g

Semisweet Dipping Chocolate (for Candy)

1 c.	nonfat dry-milk powder	250 mL
⅓ c.	unsweetened cocoa	90 mL
2 T.	grated paraffin wax	30 mL
½ c.	water	250 mL
1 T.	vegetable oil	15 mL
1 T.	liquid fructose	15 mL

Combine milk powder, cocoa, and wax in a food processor or blender; process or blend to a soft powder. Transfer into the top of a double boiler and add the water, stirring to blend. Add vegetable oil. Place over hot (not boiling) water. Cook and stir until wax pieces are completely melted and mixture is thick, smooth, and creamy. Remove double boiler from heat. Stir in liquid fructose. Allow to cool slightly. Dip candies according to recipe in cookbook or your recipe. Shake off excess chocolate. Place on very lightly greased waxed paper, and allow candies to cool completely. (If candies cannot be removed easily, slightly warm a cookie sheet in the oven, lay the waxed paper with candies on warmed cookie sheet, and remove them. Store in cool place.)

Yield: 1 c. (250 mL)
Exchange, full recipe: 3 low-fat milk
Calories, full recipe: 427
Carbohydrates, full recipe: 30 g

Chocolate Crunch Candy

1 c.	nonfat dry-milk powder	250 mL
½ c.	unsweetened cocoa powder	125 mL
2 T.	liquid fructose	30 mL
3 T.	water	45 mL
1½ c.	chow mein noodles	375 mL

Combine milk powder and cocoa in a food processor or blender. Process or blend to a fine powder. Stir in liquid fructose and water. Beat until smooth and creamy. Sightly crush the chow mein noodles, and fold them into the chocolate mixture. Drop by teaspoonfuls onto waxed paper. Cool to room temperature.

Yield: 30 pieces
Exchange, 1 piece: ⅕ bread
Calories, 1 piece: 11
Carbohydrates, 1 piece: 3 g

Fudge Candy

13-oz. can	evaporated skim milk	385-mL can
3 T.	unsweetened cocoa powder	45 mL
¼ c.	butter	60 mL
1 T.	granulated fructose	15 mL
dash	salt	dash
1 t.	vanilla extract	5 mL
2½ c.	unsweetened cereal crumbs	625 mL
¼ c.	nuts, chopped very fine	60 mL

Combine milk and cocoa in a saucepan. Cook and beat over low heat until cocoa is dissolved. Add butter, fructose, salt, and vanilla. Bring to a boil. Reduce heat and cook for 2 minutes. Remove from heat; add cereal crumbs and work in with a wooden spoon. Cool 15 minutes. Divide dough in half; roll each half into an 8-in. (20-cm)-long tube. Roll each tube in the finely chopped nuts. Wrap in waxed paper, and chill overnight. Cut into ¼-in. (8-mm) slices.

Yield: 64 candies
Exchange, 1 candy: ¼ bread, ¼ fat
Calories, 1 candy: 30
Carbohydrates, 1 candy: 4 g

Fruit Candy Bars

1 env.	unflavored gelatin	1 env.
¼ c.	cold water	60 mL
1 c.	dried apricots	250 mL
1 c.	raisins	250 mL
1 c.	pecans	250 mL
1 T.	all-purpose flour	15 mL
2 T.	grated orange peel	30 mL
1 t.	rum extract	5 mL

Sprinkle gelatin over water in a saucepan; allow to soften for 5 minutes. Heat and stir until gelatin is completely dissolved. Meanwhile, combine apricots, raisins, pecans, flour, and orange peel in a blender or food processor. Blend or process until finely chopped. Add fruit mixture to dissolved gelatin. Add rum extract and stir to completely blend. Line an 8-in. (20-cm)-square pan with plastic wrap or waxed paper. Spread fruit mixture evenly in the bottom of the pan. Set aside to cool completely so that candy is firm. Turn out onto a cutting board; then cut into 24 bars and wrap individually.

Yield: 24 bars
Exchange, 1 bar: 1 fruit, ½ fat
Calories, 1 bar: 68
Carbohydrates, 1 bar: 17 g

Coconut Macaroons

1 c.	evaporated skim milk	250 mL
2 t.	granulated fructose	10 mL
3 c.	unsweetened shredded coconut	750 mL

Combine milk and fructose in large bowl. Stir until fructose is dissolved. Add coconut and stir until coconut is completely moistened. Drop by teaspoonfuls onto greased cookie sheets, 2 to 3 in. (5 to 7 cm) apart. Bake at 350 °F (175 °C) for 15 minutes or until tops are lightly browned. Remove from pan immediately.

Yield: 48 candies
Exchange, 1 candy: ⅕ fruit, ½ fat
Calories, 1 candy: 31
Carbohydrates, 1 candy: 2 g

Butter Rum Candy

5 c.	unsweetened puffed rice	1250 mL
3 T.	granulated fructose	45 mL
2	egg whites	2
2 t.	butter rum flavoring	10 mL
1 t.	vanilla extract	5 mL

Pour rice into blender and work into a powder. Pour into a large bowl or food processor. Add remaining ingredients. Work with wooden spoon or steel blade until mixture is completely blended (mixture will be sticky). Form into 20 patties. Place patties on an ungreased cookie sheet. Bake at 300 °F (150 °C) for 20 minutes or until surface of patties feels dry.

Yield: 20 candies
Exchange, 1 candy: ⅕ bread
Calories, 1 candy: 23
Carbohydrates, 1 candy: 3 g

Marshmallow Crème

3 env.	unflavored gelatin	3 env.
¼ c.	cold water	60 mL
¾ c.	boiling water	190 mL
3 T.	granulated fructose	45 mL
1 t.	white vanilla extract	5 mL
3	egg whites	3

Sprinkle gelatin over cold water in a mixing bowl; set aside for 5 minutes to allow gelatin to soften. Add to boiling water in a saucepan; cook and stir until gelatin is dissolved. Remove from heat. Cool to consistency of thick syrup. Stir in fructose and vanilla. Beat egg whites into soft peaks. Very slowly trickle a small stream of gelatin mixture into egg whites, beating until all gelatin mixture is blended. Continue beating until light and fluffy. Pour into prepared pan.

For marshmallows: Fill a 13 × 9 × 2 in. (33 × 23 × 5 cm) pan with flour or cornstarch to desired depth. Form "moulds" with a small glass, inside of dough cutter, or object of desired size by pressing form into flour to the bottom of the pan. Spoon marshmallow crème into mould and refrigerate until set. Dust or roll tops of marshmallows in flour; shake off excess. Keep refrigerated.

Optional marshmallows: Lightly grease and flour 13 × 9 in. (33 × 23 cm) baking pan. Pour marshmallow crème in pan, spreading out evenly. Refrigerate until set and cut to desired size.

Yield: 4 c. (1000 mL)
Exchange, 1 c. (250 mL): negligible
Calories, 1 c. (250 mL): negligible
Carbohydrates, 1 c. (250 mL): negligible

Sweetened Citrus Peel

1 c.	water	250 mL
¼ t.	Stevia Rebaudiana extract	1 mL
⅓ c.	thin peel of any citrus fruit (cut in matchstick-sized strips)	90 mL

Combine water and Stevia Rebaudiana in a saucepan. Stir to dissolve powder. Cook over medium heat until just boiling. Reduce heat, add citrus peel, and simmer for 15 minutes. Let cool to room temperature. Cover and refrigerate at least 6 to 8 hours or overnight. Drain peel thoroughly and mince. Use as garnish on desserts.

Yield: 2 T (30 mL)
Exchange: negligible
Calories: negligible
Carbohydrates: negligible

Sauces

Rhubarb Sauce

1 lb.	fresh or frozen rhubarb	454 g
¾ c.	water	190 mL
1 t.	cornstarch	5 mL
¼ c.	cold water	60 mL
2 T.	liquid Stevia Rebaudiana extract (page 8)	30 mL
	or	
¾ c.	granulated sugar replacement	190 mL
dash	salt (optional)	dash

Combine rhubarb and the ¾ c. (190 mL) of water in a saucepan or microwavable bowl. Cook until rhubarb is tender, stirring occasionally. Or microwave on HIGH for 2 minutes; then reduce to MEDIUM until rhubarb is tender (about 6 to 7 minutes). Dissolve cornstarch in the ¼ c. (60 mL) of cold water. Stir into rhubarb mixture. Stir in the sweetener of your choice. If desired, add the dash of salt. Cook and stir until mixture has lost its cloudy look. Serve warm or chilled.

Yield: 6 servings
Exchange, 1 serving: negligible
Calories, 1 serving: negligible
Carbohydrates, 1 serving: negligible

Orange Cranberry Sauce

1 pkg. (12-oz.)	fresh cranberries, cleaned	1 pkg. (340-g)
⅛ t.	Stevia Rebaudiana extract	½ mL
	or	
½ c.	granulated fructose	125 mL
½ c.	orange-juice concentrate, undiluted	125 mL

Combine all ingredients in a saucepan. Cook until mixture comes to a boil, stirring occasionally. Reduce heat and boil gently until all cranberries have "popped." Serve warm or chilled.

Yield: 6 servings, with Stevia Rebaudiana
Exchange, 1 serving: negligible
Calories, 1 serving: negligible
Carbohydrates, 1 serving: negligible

Yield: 6 servings, with granulated fructose
Exchange, 1 serving: 1 fruit
Calories, 1 serving: 64
Carbohydrates, 1 serving: 16 g

Blackberry Sauce

1-lb. pkg.	frozen, unsweetened blackberries, thawed	453-g pkg.
1 T.	all-natural orange marmalade	15 mL
1 t.	fresh lemon juice	5 mL
2 env.	aspartame sweetener	2 env.

Combine all ingredients in a food processor or blender. Process or blend into a puree. Strain sauce through a fine sieve to remove seeds. Transfer to a serving bowl. Cover and refrigerate.

Yield: 4 servings
Exchange, 1 serving: 1 fruit
Calories, 1 serving: 54
Carbohydrates, 1 serving: 15 g

Strawberry Sauce

1 qt.	fresh or unsweetened frozen strawberries, thawed	1 L
3 env.	aspartame sweetener	3 env.
1 t.	orange juice	5 mL
1 t.	fresh lemon juice	5 mL

Combine all ingredients in a food processor or blender. Process or blend into a puree. Transfer to a serving bowl. Cover and refrigerate.

Yield: 4 servings
Exchange, 1 serving: 1 fruit
Calories, 1 serving: 52
Carbohydrates, 1 serving: 13 g

Raspberry Sauce

12-oz. pkg.	frozen, unsweetened red raspberries	340-g pkg.
½ t.	cornstarch	2 mL
5 env.	aspartame sweetener	5 env.

Thaw raspberries. Transfer raspberries and their juice to a saucepan. Stir in the cornstarch. Cook over medium heat until mixture comes to a full boil and the mixture is clear. Remove from heat. Cool until you can place your hand comfortably on the bottom of the pan. Stir in the aspartame sweetener. Serve warm or chilled.

Yield: 6 servings
Exchange, 1 serving: ⅔ fruit
Calories, 1 serving: 43
Carbohydrates, 1 serving: 9 g

Brandy Sauce

1 c.	cool water	250 mL
2 t.	cornstarch	10 mL
2 T.	granulated sugar replacement	30 mL
	or	
6 env.	aspartame sweetener	6 env.
	or	
¾ t.	liquid Stevia Rebaudiana extract (page 8)	4 mL
¾ t.	brandy extract	4 mL

In a saucepan, dissolve the cornstarch in the cool water. Bring to a boil. Reduce heat and boil gently for 5 minutes. Remove from heat, and cool slightly. Stir in desired sweetener and the brandy extract. If desired, tint a light shade of brown with food coloring. This is a good sauce to use on top of the Cinnamon Apple Cheesecake (page 54).

Yield, 1 c. (250 mL)
Exchange, full recipe: negligible
Calories, full recipe: negligible
Carbohydrates, full recipe: negligible

Apricot Lemon Sauce

1 c.	apricot nectar	250 mL
1 T.	cornstarch	15 mL
3 T.	fresh lemon juice	45 mL
1 t.	grated lemon peel	5 mL
2 env.	aspartame sweetener	2 env.

Combine apricot nectar and cornstarch in a small saucepan. Stir to dissolve cornstarch. Bring to a boil. Cook and stir until mixture is smooth and thick. Stir in lemon juice and lemon peel. Remove from heat. Allow to cool until pan can be set comfortably on the palm of your hand. Stir in aspartame sweetener. This sauce is especially good for fresh berries or on plain cake.

Yield: 4 servings
Exchange, 1 serving: 1 fruit
Calories, 1 serving: 59
Carbohydrates, 1 serving: 14 g

Custard Sauce

3	egg yolks	3
2 T.	granulated sugar replacement	30 mL
dash	salt	dash
1 c.	skim milk	250 mL
½ t.	vanilla extract	2 mL
1 c.	prepared nondairy whipped topping	250 mL

Slightly beat egg yolks. Combine the beaten egg yolks with the sugar replacement and salt in a saucepan. Gradually stir in the skim milk. Cook and stir over low heat until mixture thickens and coats the spoon. Remove from heat and pour into a bowl. Stir in the vanilla. Chill thoroughly. Fold in the nondairy whipped topping.

Yield: 8 servings
Exchange, 1 serving: ½ low-fat milk
Calories, 1 serving: 57
Carbohydrates, 1 serving: 3 g

Toasted-Coconut Sauce

½ c.	unsweetened, grated coconut	125 mL
1 c.	skim milk	250 mL
2 t.	cornstarch	10 mL
½ t.	vanilla extract	2 mL
½ t.	coconut flavoring	2 mL
3 env.	aspartame sweetener	3 env.

Place coconut in a small nonstick saucepan over medium heat. Cook and stir until all the coconut is a dark tan. Combine milk and cornstarch in a measuring cup or bowl. Stir to dissolve cornstarch. Pour into toasted coconut. Continue cooking over medium heat until mixture just begins to thicken. Pour mixture through a fine sieve into a bowl to remove coconut. Return coconut liquid to the saucepan. Cook and stir until mixture is thickened to a light syrup. Remove from heat. Stir in vanilla and coconut flavoring. Cool until pan can comfortably be placed in the palm of your hand. Stir in aspartame sweetener.

Yield: 4 servings
Exchange, 1 serving: ½ low-fat milk
Calories, 1 serving: 63
Carbohydrates, 1 serving: 6 g

Glazes & Frostings

Egg-White Sweet Wash

1	egg white	1
⅛ t. (scant)	Stevia Rebaudiana extract	½ mL (scant)
	or	
⅓ c.	granulated sugar replacement	90 mL

If using Stevia Rebaudiana: Combine egg white and Stevia in a small mixing bowl, beat to soft peaks, and then brush on desired surface. If using sugar replacement: Beat egg white to very soft peaks, beat in sugar replacement, and then brush on desired surface.

Yield: enough for large coffee cake or 12 to 18 rolls
Exchange: negligible
Calories: negligible
Carbohydrates: negligible

Frosting Glaze

¼ c.	sugar-free white frosting mix	60 mL
7 t.	boiling water	35 mL

Combine the frosting mix and boiling water in a small narrow bowl or cup. Beat with a small wire whisk or fork until mixture is smooth. Dampen a pastry brush, and brush glaze over desired surface.

Yield: enough for large coffee cake or 12 to 18 rolls
Exchange: negligible
Calories: negligible
Carbohydrates: negligible

Egg-Yolk Glaze

1	egg yolk	1
2 T.	water	30 mL

Beat egg yolk and water until light and fluffy. Brush on desired surface.

Yield: enough for large coffee cake or 12 to 18 rolls
Exchange: negligible
Calories: negligible
Carbohydrates: negligible

Frosting Drizzle

2 t.	skim milk	30 mL
½ c.	sugar-free white frosting mix	152 mL

Pour milk into a small bowl, cup, or custard cup. Heat in microwave until boiling. Gradually add the frosting mix, 1 T. (15 mL) at a time, while constantly whipping with a fork or small wire whisk. Place in refrigerator and chill thoroughly. Drizzle on desired surface.

Yield: enough for large coffee cake or 12 to 18 rolls
Exchange: negligible
Calories: negligible
Carbohydrates: negligible

Powdered-Fructose Icing or Filling

8 T.	Powdered Fructose (opposite page)	120 mL
½ t.	vanilla extract	2 mL
1 T.	plain low-fat yogurt	15 mL
1	egg white	1

Combine powdered fructose, vanilla, and yogurt in a small bowl. Beat to blend. Beat egg white to firm peaks. Very slowly add fructose mixture to beaten egg white.

Yield: 10 servings
Exchange, 1 serving: 1 fruit
Calories, 1 serving: 53
Carbohydrates, 1 serving: 7 g

Powdered-Sugar Replacement

½ c.	nonfat dry-milk powder	125 mL
½ c.	cornstarch	125 mL
¼ c.	granulated sugar replacement	60 mL

Combine all ingredients in a blender. Process on HIGH until powdered.

Yield: 1 c. (250 mL)
Exchange, ¼ c. (60 mL): ½ skim milk, ½ bread
Calories, ¼ c. (60 mL): 81
Carbohydrates, ¼ c. (60 mL): 13 g

Powdered Fructose

| 1 c. | granulated fructose | 250 ml |
| ⅓ c. | cornstarch | 90 mL |

Combine fructose and cornstarch in a blender container. Process on HIGH for 30 to 45 seconds or until mixture appears like powdered sugar. Do not overprocess or mixture will become liquid and sticky.

Yield: 24 T. (360 mL)
Exchange, 1 T. (15 mL): 1 fruit
Calories, 1 T. (15 mL): 62
Carbohydrates, 1 T. (15 mL): 8 g

Sweetened Whipped Topping

| 1 c. | prepared nondairy whipped topping | 250 mL |
| 1 T. | Powdered Fructose (above) | 15 mL |

Stir fructose into nondairy whipped topping. Refrigerate until ready to use.

Yield: 1 c. (250 mL) or 16 servings
Exchange, 1 serving: negligible
Calories, 1 serving: negligible
Carbohydrates, 1 serving: negligible

Chocolate-Flavored Nondairy Whipped Topping

1 env.	nondairy whipped-topping powder (to yield 2 c. [500 mL])	1 env.
1½ T.	granulated sugar replacement	21 mL
	or	
2 t.	granulated fructose	10 mL
2 T.	unsweetened cocoa powder	30 mL
½ c.	cold skim milk	125 mL

Combine all ingredients in a narrow bowl. Beat until thick and fluffy.

Yield: 2 c. (500 mL) or 10 servings, such as frosting on a cake
Exchange, 1 serving: ½ fat
Calories, 1 serving: 36
Carbohydrates, 1 serving: negligible

Yield: 20 servings, used as free-food garnish
Exchange, 1 T. (15 mL): negligible
Calories, 1 T.: negligible
Carbohydrates, 1 T.: negligible

From the Kitchen of . . .

The recipes that follow are reprinted with permission of Bernard Food Industries, Inc. and Featherweight Foods.

From the Kitchen of Bernard

Anise Cookies

1 box	Sweet 'n Low brand lemon cake mix
3 T.	water
¼ to ½ t.	anise extract (depending on flavor intensity desired)
¼ c.	finely chopped almonds

Combine all ingredients in mixing bowl. Mix 3 minutes. Drop by level teaspoons onto lightly greased or foil-lined baking sheet. Bake at 350 °F for 10 to 12 minutes.

Makes 6 dozen small cookies—15 calories per cookie.

Blueberry Cupcakes

1 box	Sweet 'n Low brand white cake mix
⅔ c.	water
¾ c.	blueberries, unsweetened (fresh, canned, or frozen)*

*Drain canned blueberries, or thaw frozen blueberries.

Mix half the water with cake mix for 3 minutes, using mixer. Add the balance of water and mix 1 minute. Pour batter into 10 muffin cups (paper or foil). Drop a spoon of berries on top of each. Bake at 375 °F for 20 minutes.

Makes 10 cupcakes—97 calories per cupcake.

Brownies

1 box	Sweet 'n Low brand chocolate cake mix
¼ t.	salt (omit if sodium-restricted)
1 c.	water
1 t.	vanilla extract
¼ c.	chopped almonds

Mix cake mix, salt, ¼ c. water, and vanilla extract in mixer for 3 minutes. Gradually add balance of water and mix 1 minute. Pour batter into lightly greased 10-in.-square baking pan. (One 8-in.-square and one 8 × 4-in. pan can be used instead.) Sprinkle batter with chopped almonds. Bake at 375 °F for 25 minutes. Cut bars in pan.

Makes 2 dozen bars, 2½ × 1½ in.—45 calories per brownie.

Banana Date Nut Bars

1	small ripe banana (⅓ c.) mashed
1 box	Sweet 'n Low brand banana cake mix
¾ c.	water
½ c.	chopped dates (16 dates)
¼ c.	chopped pecans

Mash small banana in mixing bowl. Add cake mix and ¼ c. water. Mix 3 minutes. Add balance of water and mix 1 minute. Pour batter into lightly greased 10-in.-square baking pan. (One 8-in.-square and one 8 × 4-in. pan can be used instead.) Sprinkle batter with ½ c. chopped dates and ¼ c. chopped pecans. Bake at 375 °F for 30 minutes or until done. Cut bars in pan.

Makes 2 dozen bars, 2½ × 1½ in.—58 calories per bar.

Prune Walnut Bars

1 box	Sweet 'n Low brand lemon cake mix
1 c.	water
½ c.	chopped, dried, pitted prunes (10 prunes)
¼ c.	chopped walnuts

Mix cake mix and ¼ c. water in mixer for 3 minutes. Gradually add remaining water and mix 1 minute. Pour batter into lightly greased 10-

in.-square pan. (One 8-in.-square and one 8 × 4-in. pan can be used instead.) Sprinkle chopped prunes and chopped walnuts over the batter. Bake at 375 °F for 30 minutes. Cut bars in pan. Cool thoroughly before storing or serving.

Makes 2 dozen bars, 2½ × 1½ in.—45 calories per bar.

Marble Cake

1 box	Sweet 'n Low brand white cake mix
⅔ c.	water
2 T.	cocoa (unsweetened)

Mix half the water with cake mix for 3 minutes, using mixer. Add the balance of water and mix 1 minute. Pour 1⅓ c. of this white batter into lightly greased and wax paper–lined pen. Use either 8-in. square, 8-in. round, or 8 × 4 in. loaf pan. Sift the cocoa into remaining white batter and mix until well blended. Spoon chocolate batter on top of white batter. Zigzag knife through to marble batter. Bake at 375 °F for 25 minutes for round or square cake, and for 35 to 40 minutes for loaf cake. Cool slightly before removing from pan.

Makes 10 servings—95 calories per serving.

Mocha-Crème Dessert Crepes

1 box	Sweet 'n Low brand pancake and crepe mix, plus water
	low-calorie whipped-topping mix, to make 2 pts., plus water and vanilla
1 t.	instant-coffee granules
2 T.	sifted cocoa, unsweetened
4 t.	shaved chocolate, dietetic

Using entire box of pancake and crepe mix, prepare 16 crepes according to directions on package. Mix topping mix, coffee granules, and cocoa in mixing bowl. Add water and vanilla according to topping-mix directions. Set crepes in muffin cups or roll like cones. Fill each crepe with ¼ c. mocha-crème mixture. Garnish each with ¼ t. shaved chocolate.

Makes 16 crepes—107 calories per crepe.

Mocha Torte

Cake:

1 box	Sweet 'n Low brand chocolate cake mix
¼ t.	salt
¾ c.	water

Filling and topping:

1 c.	low-calorie whipped topping
¼ t.	instant-coffee granules
1½ t.	sifted cocoa, unsweetened
1 t.	shaved chocolate, dietetic

Cake: Mix cake mix and salt with half the water for 3 minutes in mixer. Add the balance of water and mix 1 minute. Pour batter into lightly greased and wax paper–lined 8 × 4 in. loaf pan. Bake at 375 °F 35 to 40 minutes. Cool slightly before removing from pan. Cool thoroughly before slicing horizontally into three layers.

Filling and Topping: Flavor low-calorie whipped topping with coffee granules and cocoa. Spread ¼ c. topping over each layer (including top layer) and the remaining ¼ c. on the sides of the loaf after the layers are stacked. Garnish top of torte with 1 t. of shaved chocolate. Refrigerate until serving time.

Makes one 8 × 4 in. torte, 10 servings—105 calories per serving.

Nutmeg Cake Ring

1 box	Sweet 'n Low brand banana cake mix
⅛ t.	nutmeg
2 T.	finely chopped almonds
⅔ c.	water

Combine cake mix, nutmeg, and 1 T. chopped almonds in mixing bowl. Add half the water and mix 3 minutes. Add balance of water and mix 1 minute. Lightly grease and wax paper–line a ring mould (1-q. capacity). Sprinkle remaining T. chopped almonds on bottom of pan. Pour batter into pan. Bake at 375 °F for 25 to 30 minutes. Cool slightly. Invert onto serving plate.

Makes 10 servings—101 calories per servings.

From the Kitchen of Featherweight

Brandied-Cherry Dessert

16-oz. can	Featherweight water-pack pitted dark sweet cherries, drained (reserve liquid)
½ c.	brandy
1 pkg. (2 envs.)	Featherweight cherry gelatin
2 c.	boiling water
6 T.	Featherweight whipped topping

Combine drained cherries and brandy; set aside for about 1 hour. Empty both envelopes of gelatin into a bowl. Add boiling water and stir until dissolved. Drain cherries, reserving brandy. Combine brandy and reserved cherry liquid; add enough cold water to make 1½ c. Add to gelatin and stir in cherries. Pour into an 11 × 7 × 1½-in. dish. Chill until firm. Cut into cubes; spoon into dessert dishes. Then top each with 1 T. whipped topping.

Yield: 6 servings
Exchange, 1 serving: 2 fruit
Calories: 104

Frosty Pineapple Dessert

20-oz. can	Featherweight water-pack pineapple chunks, drained
3½ c.	chopped ice
½ t.	vanilla extract
⅙ t.	mint extract
6	mint sprigs

Add all ingredients, except mint sprigs, to a blender; cover. Blend at high speed until finely crushed. Serve in chilled dessert dishes with mint sprigs on top.

Yield: 6 servings
Exchange, 1 serving: 1 fruit
Calories, 1 serving: 50

Orange Dream Dessert

½ pkg.   Featherweight orange gelatin
(1 env.)
¼ c.   boiling water
2 c.   cold skim milk

Add gelatin and boiling water to a blender; cover. Blend at medium speed for 20 seconds. Add cold milk and blend at high speed for 20 seconds. Chill in refrigerator at least 30 minutes. Blend 1 minute at high speed. Serve immediately in chilled glasses.

Yield: 4 servings
Exchange, 1 serving: ½ milk
Calories: 55

Apricot Morning Drink

16-oz. can   Featherweight water-pack apricot halves
1½ c.   skim milk
3   eggs
1 t.   vanilla extract
½ t.   Featherweight liquid sweetener
             ground cinnamon

Add all ingredients, except cinnamon, to a blender; cover. Blend at medium speed for 30 seconds. Pour into glasses and sprinkle top of drink with cinnamon.

Yield: 3 servings
Exchange, 1 serving: 1 fruit, 1 meat, ½ milk
Calories, 1 serving: 191

Dessert-Products Information

Food manufacturers now include nutritional information on the labels of their products. This information can be very useful to anyone using the American Diabetes Association's Exchange Lists in their diets. The labels show the number of calories and the grams of protein, carbohydrates, and fat in each serving. Most of the labels resemble the following example.

NUTRITIONAL INFORMATION PER SERVING
Servings per container: 12
Serving size (Cookie): 3
Calories per serving: 170
Protein: 2 g
Carbohydrates: 22 g
Fat: 7 g

With this information, you can work out the food exchange on any product. The following exchange list is needed for calculations.

Exchange	Calories	Carbohydrates (grams)	Protein (grams)	Fat (grams)
Starch/Bread	80	15	3	trace
Meat				
Lean	55	0	7	3
Medium-fat	75	0	7	5
High-fat	100	0	7	8
Vegetable	25	5	2	0
Fruit	60	15	0	0
Milk				
Skim	90	12	8	trace
Low-fat	120	12	8	5
Whole	150	12	8	8
Fat	45	0	0	5

Compare the nutrient value on the label with the nutrient value on the exchange list. Count whole and nearest half exchanges.

	Exchange	C	P	F
1. List the grams of carbohydrates, protein, and fat per serving.		22	2	7
2. Subtract carbohydrates first. Bread exchange has 15 g carbohydrates + 3 g protein	1 bread	−15	−3	
		7	−1	7
3. Think about the ingredients in a cookie and compare the next-nearest carbohydrate exchange. Fruit has 15 g; ½ fruit has 7.5 or 7.	½ fruit	−7		
		0	−1	7
4. Compare the fat exchange.	1 fat			−5
			−1	2

You have 2 grams of fat left, or approximately ½ fat exchange; therefore, your exchange on 1 serving of this product is equivalent to 1 bread, ½ fruit, and 1½ fat.

5. Check with calories

    1 bread = 80 calories
    ½ fruit = 30 calories
    1½ fat = 67 calories

Total: 177 calories (Product Information states 170)

It's important to realize that most exchanges figured on foods will vary because the averages are used for calculating the original exchange value.

Product Lists

The product lists that follow are reprinted with permission of Weight Watchers, Featherweight Foods, Flavorland Foods, Health Valley Foods, Pepperidge Farm, and Kemp.

Remember these are only general reference lists. Many of the products' ingredients vary from area to area, and from season to season. You need to check the products' labels for the most recently updated information.

Weight Watchers Products

Cheesecake
Serving size: 3.9 oz.
Bread: ½
Meat: ½ lean
Fruit: 1
Fat: 1
Milk: ½ skim

Strawberry Cheesecake
Serving size: 3.9 oz.
Bread: ½
Meat: ½ lean
Fruit: 1
Fat: ½
Milk: ½ skim

Brownie Cheesecake*
Serving size: 3.5 oz.
Bread: ½
Meat: ½ lean
Fruit: 1
Fat: ½
Milk: ½ skim

Carrot Cake*
Serving size: 3 oz.
Bread: 1
Vegetables: 1
Fruit: ½
Fat: 1

Chocolate Cake*
Serving size: 2.5 oz.
Bread: 2
Fat: 1

Black Forest Cake*
Serving size: 3 oz.
Bread: 1
Fruit: 1
Fat: 1

Double Fudge Cake*
Serving size: 2.75 oz.
Bread: 1½
Fruit: 1
Fat: 1

German Chocolate Cake*
Serving size: 2.5 oz.
Bread: 1
Fruit: 1
Fat: 1½

Cherries and Cream Cake*
Serving size: 3 oz.
Bread: 1
Fruit: 1
Fat: 1

*This product contains more than 5 percent carbohydrate calories from refined sugars. Consult with your dietitian for information on if or how often these may be included in your diet.

Boston Cream Pie*
Serving size: 3 oz.
Bread: ½
Fruit: 1½
Fat: ½
Milk: ½ skim

Chocolate Mocha Pie*
Serving size: 2.75 oz.
Bread: ½
Fruit: ½
Fat: 1
Milk: ½ skim

Chocolate Brownie*
Serving size: 1.25 oz.
Bread: ½
Fruit: ½
Fat: ½

Chocolate Mousse*
Serving size: 2.5 oz.
Bread: 1
Fat: 1
Milk: ½ skim

Apple Pie*
Serving size: 3.5 oz.
Bread: ½
Fruit: 2
Fat: 1

Apple Crisp*
Serving size: 3.5 oz.
Bread: 1
Fruit: 1½
Fat: 1

Featherweight Products

LOW-CALORIE FRUIT SPREADS

For Strawberry, Grape, Apple, and Blackberry Jelly, and for Apricot, Blackberry, Peach, Red Raspberry, and Strawberry Preserves:
Serving size: 1 t
Calories: 4
Protein: 0 g
Carbohydrates: 1 g
Fat: 0 g

LOW-CALORIE SYRUPS

For Blueberry and Pancake Syrups:
Serving size: 1 T
Calories: 16
Protein: 0 g
Carbohydrates: 4 g
Fat: 0 g

SWEETENERS

Liquid Sweetening
Serving size: 3 dps.
Calories: 0
Protein: 0 g
Carbohydrates: 0 g
Fat: 0 g

Fructose Sweetener
Serving size: 1 t
Calories: 12
Protein: 0 g
Carbohydrates: 3 g
Fat: 0 g

FRUIT

JP Apricot Halves
Serving size: ½ c
Calories: 50
Protein: 1 g
Carbohydrates: 12 g
Fat: 0 g

JP Fruit Cocktail
Serving size: ½ c.
Calories: 50
Protein: 1 g
Carbohydrates: 14 g
Fat: 0 g

JP Yellow Cling Peach Halves, Slices
Serving size: ½ c
Calories: 50
Protein: 0 g
Carbohydrates: 14 g
Fat: 0 g

WP Mandarin Oranges
Serving size: ½ c
Calories: 35
Protein: 0 g
Carbohydrates: 8 g
Fat: 0 g

JP Pear Halves
Serving size: ½ c
Calories: 60
Protein: 0 g
Carbohydrates: 15 g
Fat: 0 g

JP Pineapple Slices
Serving size: ½ c
Calories: 70
Protein: 0 g
Carbohydrates: 18 g
Fat: 0 g

WP Applesauce
Serving size: ½ c
Calories: 50
Protein: 0 g
Carbohydrates: 12 g
Fat: 0 g

JP Fruit Salad
Serving size: ½ c
Calories: 50
Protein: 1 g
Carbohydrates: 13 g
Fat: 0 g

LOW-SODIUM/LOW-CALORIE NUTRASWEET DESSERTS

For Butterscotch, Chocolate, and Vanilla Puddings:
Serving size: ½ c
Calories: 12
Protein: 0 g
Carbohydrates: 3 g
Fat: 0 g

For Raspberry, Strawberry, Cherry, Lemon, Lime, and Orange Gelatins:
Serving size: ½ c
Calories: 10
Protein: 2 g
Carbohydrates: 1 g
Fat: 0 g

For Vanilla and Butterscotch Instant Puddings:
Serving size: ½ c.
Calories: 100
Protein: 4 g
Carbohydrates: 19 g
Fat: 0 g

For Vanilla and Lemon Custards:
Serving size: ½ c
Calories: 40
Protein: 1 g
Carbohydrates: 8 g
Fat: 0 g

COOKIES

For Chocolate Chip, Double Chocolate Chip, Lemon, Vanilla, and Oatmeal Raisin Cookies:
Serving size: 1 cookie
Calories: 45
Protein: 1 g
Carbohydrates: 6 g
Fat: 2 g

For Chocolate, Vanilla, and Strawberry Creme Wafers:
Serving size: 1 wafer
Calories: 20
Protein: 0 g
Carbohydrates: .3 g
Fat: 1 g

CANDY

For Milk Chocolate and Chocolate Crunch Bars:
Serving size: 1 section
Calories: 80
Protein: 1 g
Carbohydrates: 7 g
Fat: 6 g

Caramels
Serving size: 1 piece
Calories: 30
Protein: 0 g
Carbohydrates: 5 g
Fat: 1 g

Flavorland Products

FROZEN FRUITS

Blackberries
Serving size: 4 oz.
Servings per package: 4
Calories: 70
Protein: 1 g
Carbohydrates: 18 g
Fat: 0 g

Black Raspberries
Serving size: 4 oz.
Servings per package: 3
Calories: 60
Protein: 1 g
Carbohydrates: 13 g
Fat: 1 g

Blueberries
Serving size: 4 oz.
Servings per package: 4
Calories: 60
Protein: 1 g
Carbohydrates: 14 g
Fat: 1 g

Boysenberries
Serving size: 4 oz.
Servings per package: 4
Calories: 60
Protein: 1 g
Carbohydrates: 14 g
Fat: 0 g

Deluxe Fruit Mix
Serving size: 4 oz.
Servings per package: 4
Calories: 50
Protein: 1 g
Carbohydrates: 13 g
Fat: 0 g

Dark Sweet Cherries
Serving size: 4 oz.
Servings per package: 4
Calories: 80
Protein: 1 g
Carbohydrates: 19 g
Fat: 1 g

Fruit Medley
Serving size: 4 oz.
Servings per package: 4
Calories: 60
Protein: 1 g
Carbohydrates: 14 g
Fat: 1 g

Melon Balls
Serving size: 4 oz.
Servings per package: 4
Calories: 35
Protein: 1 g
Carbohydrates: 9 g
Fat: 0 g

Peach Slices
Serving size: 4 oz.
Servings per package: 4
Calories: 50
Protein: 1 g
Carbohydrates: 13 g
Fat: 0 g

Red Raspberries
Serving size: 4 oz.
Servings per package: 3
Calories: 60
Protein: 2 g
Carbohydrates: 13 g
Fat: 0 g

Rhubarb
Serving size: 4 oz.
Servings per package: 4
Calories: 25
Protein: 1 g
Carbohydrates: 6 g
Fat: 0 g

Red Tart Cherries
Serving size: 4 oz.
Servings per package: 4
Calories: 50
Protein: 1 g
Carbohydrates: 12 g
Fat: 0 g

Whole Strawberries
Serving size: 4 oz.
Servings per package: 4
Calories: 40
Protein: 1 g
Carbohydrates: 10 g
Fat: 0 g

Health Valley Products

COOKIES

For Fat-Free Cookies—Apple Spice, Apricot Delight, Date Delight, Hawaiian Fruit, and Raisin Oatmeal:
Serving size: 3 cookies
Calories: 75
Exchanges: ½ starch
 ½ fruit

For Fancy Fruit Chunks—Apricot Almond, Date Pecan, and Tropical Fruit:
Serving size: 2 cookies
Calories; 90
Exchanges: ½ starch
 ½ fruit
 ½ fat

The Great Wheat-Free Cookie
Serving size: 2 cookies
Calories: 130
Exchanges: ½ starch
½ fruit
½ fat

For Fruit Jumbos—Almond Date, Raisin Nut, Oat Bran, and Tropical Fruit; and for Honey Jumbos— Crisp Cinnamon and Crisp Peanut Butter
Serving size: 1 cookie
Calories: 70
Exchanges: 1 starch

The Great Tofu Cookie
Serving size: 2 cookies
Calories: 90
Exchanges: ½ starch
½ fruit
½ fat

SNACK BARS

For 100% Organic Fat-Free Fruit Bars—Apple, Apricot, Date, and Raisin:
Serving size: 1 bar
Calories: 140
Exchanges: 1 starch
1 fruit

For Oat Bran Jumbo Fruit Bars— Almond & Date and Fruit & Nut:
Serving size: 1 bar
Calories: 170
Exchanges: 1 starch
½ fruit
1 fat

Pepperidge Farm Products

FROZEN PRODUCTS

Puff Pastry Sheets
Serving size: ¼ sheet
Calories: 260
Protein: 4 g
Carbohydrates: 22 g
Fat: 17 g

Puff Pastry Shells
Serving size: 1
Calories: 210
Protein: 2 g
Carbohydrates: 17 g
Fat: 15 g

COOKIES

Bordeaux
Serving size: 2 cookies
Calories: 70
Protein: 1 g
Carbohydrates: 11 g
Fat: 3 g

Zurich
Serving size: 1 cookie
Calories: 60
Protein: 1 g
Carbohydrates: 10 g
Fat: 2 g

Molasses Crisp
Serving size: 2 cookies
Calories: 70
Protein: 1 g
Carbohydrates: 8 g
Fat: 3 g

Apricot Raspberry/Strawberry
Serving size: 2 cookies
Calories: 100
Protein: 1 g
Carbohydrates: 15 g
Fat: 4 g (strawberry: 5 g)

Chantilly
Serving size: 1 cookie
Calories: 80
Protein: 1 g
Carbohydrates: 14 g
Fat: 2 g

Ginger Man
Serving size: 2 cookies
Calories: 70
Protein: 1 g
Carbohydrates: 10 g
Fat: 3 g

Orleans
Serving size: 3 cookies
Calories: 90
Protein: 0 g
Carbohydrates: 11 g
Fat: 6 g

CAKES

Cherry Cake Supreme
Serving size: 3¼ oz.
Calories: 170
Protein: 0 g
Carbohydrates: 38 g
Fat: 2 g
Diet exchange: 1 starch
        1 fruit
        ½ fat

Lemon Cake Supreme
Serving size: 2¾ oz.
Calories: 170
Protein: 4 g
Carbohydrates: 26 g
Fat: 5 g
Diet exchange: 1½ starch
        1 fat

Raspberry Vanilla Swirl
Serving size: 3¼ oz.
Calories: 160
Protein: 4 g
Carbohydrates: 25 g
Fat: 5 g
Diet exchange: 1 starch
        ½ fruit
        1 fat

Chocolate Mousse Cake
Serving size: 2½ oz.
Calories: 190
Protein: 3 g
Carbohydrates: 25 g
Fat: 9 g
Diet exchange: 1½ starch
        2 fat

Strawberry Shortcake
Serving size: 3 oz.
Calories: 170
Protein: 2 g
Carbohydrates: 30 g
Fat: 5 g
Diet exchange: 1½ starch
        1 fat

Apple'n Spice Bake
Serving size: 4¼ oz.
Calories: 170
Protein: 2 g
Carbohydrates: 37 g
Fat: 2 g
Diet exchange: 1 starch
        1 fruit
        ½ fat

Kemp Novelty Products

Twin Pops (orange assorted)
Serving size: 2.5 oz.
Calories: 55
Protein: 0
Carbohydrates: 14 g
Fat: 0

Bomb Pop Jr.'s
Serving size: 2 oz.
Calories: 46
Protein: 0
Carbohydrates: 11 g
Fat: 0

Fudge Bar
Serving size: 2.5 oz.
Calories: 90
Protein: 2 g
Carbohydrates: 18 g
Fat: 0

Orange Cream Bar
Serving size: 2.5 oz.
Calories: 80
Protein: 1 g
Carbohydrates: 13 g
Fat: 2 g

Ice Cream Bar
Serving size: 2.5 oz.
Calories: 160
Protein: 1 g
Carbohydrates: 12 g
Fat: 12 g

Frozen Yogurt on a Stick (raspberry)
Serving size: 1.75 oz.
Calories: 60
Protein: 1 g
Carbohydrates: 11 g
Fat: 1 g

Frozen Yogurt Dipped on a Stick (vanilla)
Serving size: 1.75 oz.
Calories: 120
Protein: 2 g
Carbohydrates: 14 g
Fat: 7 g

Lite Pops
Serving size: 1.75 oz.
Calories: 12 g
Protein: 0
Carbohydrates: 3 g
Fat: 0

Lite Fudge Jr.'s
Serving size: 1.75 oz.
Calories: 55
Protein: 2 g
Carbohydrates: 8 g
Fat: 0

Lite Ice Milk Jr.s
Serving size: 1.75 oz.
Calories: 90
Protein: 1 g
Carbohydrates: 10 g
Fat: 5 g

Krunch Bar
Serving size: 2.2 oz.
Calories: 150
Protein: 2 g
Carbohydrates: 12 g
Fat: 11 g

Ice Cream Cup Jr.'s (Vanilla)
Serving size: 3 oz.
Calories: 100
Protein: 2 g
Carbohydrates: 12 g
Fat: 5 g

EXCHANGE LISTS

The reason for dividing food into six different groups is that foods vary in their carbohydrate, protein, fat, and calorie content. Each exchange list contains foods that are alike – each choice contains about the same amount of carbohydrate, protein, fat, and calories.

The following chart shows the amount of these nutrients in one serving from each exchange list.

Exchange List	Carbohydrate (grams)	Protein (grams)	Fat (grams)	Calories
Starch/Bread	15	3	trace	80
Meat				
Lean	–	7	3	55
Medium-Fat	–	7	5	75
High-Fat	–	7	8	100
Vegetable	5	2	–	25
Fruit	15	–	–	60
Milk				
Skim	12	8	trace	90
Lowfat	12	8	5	120
Whole	12	8	8	150
Fat	–	–	5	45

As you read the exchange lists, you will notice that one choice often is a larger amount of food than another choice from the same list. Because foods are so different, each food is measured or weighed so the amount of carbohydrate, protein, fat, and calories is the same in each choice.

You will notice symbols on some foods in the exchange groups. Foods that are high in fiber (3 grams or more per exchange) have this 🌾 symbol. High-fiber foods are good for you. It is important to eat more of these foods.

Foods that are high in sodium (400 milligrams or more of sodium per exchange) have this 🥓 symbol; foods that have 400 mg or more of sodium if two or more exchanges are eaten have this ★ symbol. It's a good idea to limit your intake of high-salt foods, especially if you have high blood pressure.

If you have a favorite food that is not included in any of these groups, ask your dietitian about it. That food can probably be worked into your meal plan, at least now and then.

The Exchange Lists are the basis of a meal-planning system designed by a committee of the American Diabetes Association and the American Dietetic Association. While designed primarily for people with diabetes and others who must follow special diets, the Exchange Lists are based on principles of good nutrition that apply to everyone. © 1989 American Diabetes Association, American Dietetic Association.

1
STARCH/BREAD LIST

E ach item in this list contains approximately 15 grams of carbohydrate, 3 grams of protein, a trace of fat, and 80 calories. Whole grain products average about 2 grams of fiber per exchange. Some foods are higher in fiber. Those foods that contain 3 or more grams of fiber per exchange are identified with the fiber symbol 🌾.

You can choose your starch exchanges from any of the items on this list. If you want to eat a starch food that is not on this list, the general rule is that:

- 1/2 cup of cereal, grain or pasta is one exchange
- 1 ounce of a bread product is one exchange

Your dietitian can help you be more exact.

CEREALS/GRAINS/PASTA

🌾 Bran cereals, concentrated (such as Bran Buds® All Bran®)	1/3 cup
🌾 Bran cereals, flaked	1/2 cup
Bulgur (cooked)	1/2 cup
Cooked cereals	1/2 cup
Cornmeal (dry)	2 1/2 Tbsp.
Grape-Nuts®	3 Tbsp.
Grits (cooked)	1/2 cup
Other ready-to-eat unsweetened cereals	3/4 cup
Pasta (cooked)	1/2 cup
Puffed cereal	1 1/2 cup
Rice, white or brown (cooked)	1/3 cup
Shredded wheat	1/2 cup
🌾 Wheat germ	3 Tbsp.

DRIED BEANS/PEAS/LENTILS

🌾 Beans and peas (cooked) (such as kidney, white, split, blackeye)	1/3 cup
🌾 Lentils (cooked)	1/3 cup
🌾 Baked beans	1/4 cup

STARCHY VEGETABLES

🌾 Corn	1/2 cup
🌾 Corn on cob, 6 in. long	1
🌾 Lima beans	1/2 cup

🌾 Peas, green (canned or frozen)	1/2 cup
🌾 Plantain	1/2 cup
Potato, baked	1 small (3 oz.)
Potato, mashed	1/2 cup
🌾 Squash, winter (acorn, butternut)	1 cup
Yam, sweet potato, plain	1/3 cup

BREAD

Bagel	1/2 (1 oz.)
Bread sticks, crisp, 4 in. long × 1/2 in.	2 (2/3 oz.)
Croutons, lowfat	1 cup
English muffin	1/2
Frankfurter or hamburger bun	1/2 (1 oz.)
Pita, 6 in. across	1/2
Plain roll, small	1 (1 oz.)
Raisin, unfrosted	1 slice (1 oz.)
Rye, pumpernickel	1 slice (1 oz.)
Tortilla, 6 in. across	1
White (including French, Italian)	1 slice (1 oz.)
Whole wheat	1 slice (1 oz.)

🌾 3 grams or more of fiber per exchange

CRACKERS/SNACKS

Animal crackers	8
Graham crackers, 2 1/2 in. square	3
Matzoh	3/4 oz.
Melba toast	5 slices
Oyster crackers	24
Popcorn (popped, no fat added)	3 cups
Pretzels	3/4 oz.
🌾 Rye crisp, 2 in. × 3 1/2 in.	4
Saltine-type crackers	6
🌾 Whole-wheat crackers, no fat added (crisp breads, such as Finn®, Kavli®, Wasa®)	2-4 slices (3/4 oz.)
Taco shell, 6 in. across	2
Waffle, 4 1/2 in. square	1
🌾 Whole-wheat crackers, fat added (such as Triscuit®)	4-6 (1 oz.)

STARCH FOODS PREPARED WITH FAT

(Count as 1 starch/bread exchange, plus 1 fat exchange.)

Biscuit, 2 1/2 in. across	1
Chow mein noodles	1/2 cup
Corn bread, 2 in. cube	1 (2 oz.)
Cracker, round butter type	6
French fried potatoes, 2 in. to 3 1/2 in. long	10 (1 1/2 oz.)
Muffin, plain, small	1
Pancake, 4 in. across	2
Stuffing, bread (prepared)	1/4 cup

2
MEAT LIST

E ach serving of meat and substitutes on this list contains about 7 grams of protein. The amount of fat and number of calories varies, depending on what kind of meat or substitute you choose. The list is divided into three parts based on the amount of fat and calories: lean meat, medium-fat meat, and high-fat meat. One ounce (one meat exchange) of each of these includes:

	Carbohydrate (grams)	Protein (grams)	Fat (grams)	Calories
Lean	0	7	3	55
Medium-Fat	0	7	5	75
High-Fat	0	7	8	100

You are encouraged to use more lean and medium-fat meat, poultry, and fish in your meal plan. This will help decrease your fat intake, which may help decrease your risk for heart disease. The items from the high-fat group are high in saturated fat, cholesterol, and calories. You should limit your choices from the high-fat group to three (3) times per week. Meat and substitutes do not contribute any fiber to your meal plan.

Meats and meat substitutes that have 400 milligrams or more of sodium per exchange are indicated with this symbol.

Meats and meat substitutes that have 400 mg or more of sodium if two or more exchanges are eaten are indicated with this symbol.

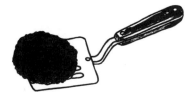

TIPS

1. Bake, roast, broil, grill, or boil these foods rather than frying them with added fat.

2. Use a nonstick pan spray or a nonstick pan to brown or fry these foods.

3. Trim off visible fat before and after cooking.

4. Do not add flour, bread crumbs, coating mixes, or fat to these foods when preparing them.

5. Weigh meat after removing bones and fat, and after cooking. Three ounces of cooked meat is about equal to 4 ounces of raw meat. Some examples of meat portions are:

   2 ounces meat (2 meat exchanges) =
      1 small chicken leg or thigh
      1/2 cup cottage cheese or tuna

   3 ounces meat (3 meat exchanges) =
      1 medium pork chop
      1 small hamburger
      1/2 of a whole chicken breast
      1 unbreaded fish fillet
      cooked meat, about the size of a deck of cards

6. Restaurants usually serve prime cuts of meat, which are high in fat and calories.

LEAN MEAT AND SUBSTITUTES
(One exchange is equal to any one of the following items.)

Beef:	USDA Select or Choice grades of lean beef, such as round, sirloin, and flank steak; tenderloin; and chipped beef 🍖	1 oz.
Pork:	Lean pork, such as fresh ham; canned, cured or boiled ham 🍖 Canadian bacon 🍖 , tenderloin.	1 oz.
Veal:	All cuts are lean except for veal cutlets (ground or cubed). Examples of lean veal are chops and roasts.	1 oz.
Poultry:	Chicken, turkey, Cornish hen (without skin)	1 oz.
Fish:	All fresh and frozen fish	1 oz.
	Crab, lobster, scallops, shrimp, clams (fresh or canned in water)	2 oz.
	Oysters	6 medium
	Tuna ★ (canned in water)	1/4 cup
	Herring ★ (uncreamed or smoked)	1 oz.
	Sardines (canned)	2 medium
Wild Game:	Venison, rabbit, squirrel	1 oz.
	Pheasant, duck, goose (without skin)	1 oz.
Cheese:	Any cottage cheese ★	1/4 cup
	Grated parmesan	2 Tbsp.
	Diet cheeses 🍖 (with less than 55 calories per ounce)	1 oz.
Other:	95% fat-free luncheon meat 🍖	1 1/2 oz.
	Egg whites	3 whites
	Egg substitutes with less than 55 calories per 1/2 cup	1/2 cup

🍖 *400 mg or more of sodium per exchange*

★ *400 mg or more of sodium if two or more exchanges are eaten*

MEDIUM-FAT MEAT AND SUBSTITUTES
(One exchange is equal to any one of the following items.)

Beef:	Most beef products fall into this category. Examples are: all ground beef, roast (rib, chuck, rump), steak (cubed, Porterhouse, T-bone), and meatloaf.	1 oz.
Pork:	Most pork products fall into this category. Examples are: chops, loin roast, Boston butt, cutlets.	1 oz.
Lamb:	Most lamb products fall into this category. Examples are: chops, leg, and roast.	1 oz.
Veal:	Cutlet (ground or cubed, unbreaded)	1 oz.
Poultry:	Chicken (with skin), domestic duck or goose (well drained of fat), ground turkey	1 oz.
Fish:	Tuna ★ (canned in oil and drained)	1/4 cup
	Salmon ★ (canned)	1/4 cup
Cheese:	Skim or part-skim milk cheeses, such as:	
	Ricotta	1/4 cup
	Mozzarella	1 oz.
	Diet cheeses 🍖 (with 56-80 calories per ounce)	1 oz.
Other:	86% fat-free luncheon meat ★	1 oz.
	Egg (high in cholesterol, limit to 3 per week)	1
	Egg substitutes with 56-80 calories per 1/4 cup	1/4 cup
	Tofu (2 1/2 in. × 2 3/4 in. × 1 in.)	4 oz.
	Liver, heart, kidney, sweetbreads (high in cholesterol)	1 oz.

🍖 *400 mg or more of sodium per exchange*

400 mg or more of sodium if two or more exchanges are eaten

HIGH-FAT MEAT AND SUBSTITUTES

Remember, these items are high in saturated fat, cholesterol, and calories, and should be used only three (3) times per week.
(One exchange is equal to any one of the following items.)

Beef:	Most USDA Prime cuts of beef, such as ribs, corned beef	1 oz.
Pork:	Spareribs, ground pork, pork sausage 🐖 (patty or link)	1 oz.
Lamb:	Patties (ground lamb)	1 oz.
Fish:	Any fried fish product	1 oz.
Cheese:	All regular cheeses, such as American 🐖, Blue 🐖, Cheddar , Monterey Jack , Swiss	1 oz.
Other:	Luncheon meat 🐖 , such as bologna, salami, pimento loaf	1 oz.
	Sausage 🐖 , such as Polish, Italian smoked	1 oz.
	Knockwurst 🐖	1 oz.
	Bratwurst	1 oz.
	Frankfurter 🐖 (turkey or chicken)	1 frank (10/lb.)
	Peanut butter (contains unsaturated fat)	1 Tbsp.

Count as one high-fat meat plus one fat exchange:

Frankfurter 🐖 (beef, pork, or combination)	1 frank (10/lb.)

🐖 *400 mg or more of sodium per exchange*

400 mg or more of sodium if two or more exchanges are eaten

3
VEGETABLE LIST

E ach vegetable serving on this list contains about 5 grams of carbohydrate, 2 grams of protein, and 25 calories.
Vegetables contain 2-3 grams of dietary fiber. Vegetables which contain 400 mg or more of sodium per exchange are identified with a 🐷 symbol.

Vegetables are a good source of vitamins and minerals. Fresh and frozen vegetables have more vitamins and less added salt. Rinsing canned vegetables will remove much of the salt.

Unless otherwise noted, the serving size for vegetables (one vegetable exchange) is:

1/2 cup of cooked vegetables or vegetable juice
1 cup of raw vegetables

Artichoke (1/2 medium)
Asparagus
Beans (green, wax, Italian)
Bean sprouts
Beets
Broccoli
Brussels sprouts
Cabbage, cooked
Carrots
Cauliflower
Eggplant
Greens (collard, mustard, turnip)
Kohlrabi
Leeks

Mushrooms, cooked
Okra
Onions
Pea pods
Peppers (green)
Rutabaga
Sauerkraut 🐷
Spinach, cooked
Summer squash (crookneck)
Tomato (one large)
Tomato/vegetable juice 🐷
Turnips
Water chestnuts
Zucchini, cooked

Starchy vegetables such as corn, peas, and potatoes are found on the Starch/Bread List.

🐷 *400 mg or more of sodium per exchange*

4
FRUIT LIST

Each item on this list contains about 15 grams of carbohydrate and 60 calories. Fresh, frozen, and dried fruits have about 2 grams of fiber per exchange. Fruits that have 3 or more grams of fiber per exchange have a ꙭ symbol. Fruit juices contain very little dietary fiber.

The carbohydrate and calorie content for a fruit exchange are based on the usual serving of the most commonly eaten fruits. Use fresh fruits or fruits frozen or canned without sugar added. Whole fruit is more filling than fruit juice and may be a better choice for those who are trying to lose weight. Unless otherwise noted, the serving size for one fruit exchange is:

1/2 cup of fresh fruit or fruit juice
1/4 cup of dried fruit

FRESH, FROZEN, AND UNSWEETENED CANNED FRUIT

Apple (raw, 2 in. across)	1 apple
Applesauce (unsweetened)	1/2 cup
Apricots (medium, raw)	4 apricots
Apricots (canned)	1/2 cup, or 4 halves
Banana (9 in. long)	1/2 banana
ꙭ Blackberries (raw)	3/4 cup
ꙭ Blueberries (raw)	3/4 cup
Cantaloupe (5 in. across)	1/3 melon
(cubes)	1 cup
Cherries (large, raw)	12 cherries
Cherries (canned)	1/2 cup
Figs (raw, 2 in. across)	2 figs
Fruit cocktail (canned)	1/2 cup
Grapefruit (medium)	1/2 grapefruit
Grapefruit (segments)	3/4 cup
Grapes (small)	15 grapes
Honeydew melon (medium)	1/8 melon
(cubes)	1 cup
Kiwi (large)	1 kiwi
Mandarin oranges	3/4 cup
Mango (small)	1/2 mango
ꙭ Nectarine (2 1/2 in. across)	1 nectarine
Orange (2 1/2 in. across)	1 orange
Papaya	1 cup
Peach (2 3/4 in. across)	1 peach, or 3/4 cup
Peaches (canned)	1/2 cup or 2 halves
Pear	1/2 large, or 1 small
Pears (canned)	1/2 cup, or 2 halves
Persimmon (medium, native)	2 persimmons
Pineapple (raw)	3/4 cup
Pineapple (canned)	1/3 cup
Plum (raw, 2 in. across)	2 plums
ꙭ Pomegranate	1/2 pomegranate
ꙭ Raspberries (raw)	1 cup
ꙭ Strawberries (raw, whole)	1 1/4 cup
ꙭ Tangerine (2 1/2 in. across)	2 tangerines
Watermelon (cubes)	1 1/4 cup

DRIED FRUIT

ꙭ Apples	4 rings
ꙭ Apricots	7 halves
Dates	2 1/2 medium
ꙭ Figs	1 1/2
ꙭ Prunes	3 medium
Raisins	2 Tbsp.

FRUIT JUICE

Apple juice/cider	1/2 cup
Cranberry juice cocktail	1/3 cup
Grapefruit juice	1/2 cup
Grape juice	1/3 cup
Orange juice	1/2 cup
Pineapple juice	1/2 cup
Prune juice	1/3 cup

ꙭ 3 or more grams of fiber per exchange

5
MILK LIST

Each serving of milk or milk products on this list contains about 12 grams of carbohydrate and 8 grams of protein. The amount of fat in milk is measured in percent (%) of butterfat. The calories vary, depending on what kind of milk you choose. The list is divided into three parts based on the amount of fat and calories: skim/very lowfat milk, lowfat milk, and whole milk. One serving (one milk exchange) of each of these includes:

	Carbohydrate (grams)	Protein (grams)	Fat (grams)	Calories
Skim/Very Lowfat	12	8	trace	90
Lowfat	12	8	5	120
Whole	12	8	8	150

Milk is the body's main source of calcium, the mineral needed for growth and repair of bones. Yogurt is also a good source of calcium. Yogurt and many dry or powdered milk products have different amounts of fat. If you have questions about a particular item, read the label to find out the fat and calorie content.

Milk is good to drink, but it can also be added to cereal, and to other foods. Many tasty dishes such as sugar-free pudding are made with milk. Add life to plain yogurt by adding one of your fruit exchanges to it.

SKIM AND VERY LOWFAT MILK

skim milk	1 cup
1/2% milk	1 cup
1% milk	1 cup
lowfat buttermilk	1 cup
evaporated skim milk	1/2 cup
dry nonfat milk	1/3 cup
plain nonfat yogurt	8 oz.

LOWFAT MILK

2% milk	1 cup fluid
plain lowfat yogurt (with added nonfat milk solids)	8 oz.

WHOLE MILK

The whole milk group has much more fat per serving than the skim and lowfat groups. Whole milk has more than 3 1/4% butterfat. Try to limit your choices from the whole milk group as much as possible.

whole milk	1 cup
evaporated whole milk	1/2 cup
whole plain yogurt	8 oz.

6

FAT LIST

Each serving on the fat list contains about 5 grams of fat and 45 calories.

The foods on the fat list contain mostly fat, although some items may also contain a small amount of protein. All fats are high in calories and should be carefully measured. Everyone should modify fat intake by eating unsaturated fats instead of saturated fats. The sodium content of these foods varies widely Check the label for sodium information.

UNSATURATED FATS

Avocado	1/8 medium
Margarine	1 tsp.
★ Margarine, diet	1 Tbsp.
Mayonnaise	1 tsp.
★ Mayonnaise, reduced-calorie	1 Tbsp.

Nuts and Seeds:

Almonds, dry roasted	6 whole
Cashews, dry roasted	1 Tbsp.
Pecans	2 whole
Peanuts	20 small or 10 large
Walnuts	2 whole
Other nuts	1 Tbsp.
Seeds, pine nuts, sun-flower (without shells)	1 Tbsp.
Pumpkin seeds	2 tsp.

Oil (corn, cottonseed, safflower, soybean, sunflower, olive, peanut)	1 tsp.
Olives	10 small or 5 large
Salad dressing, mayonnaise-type	2 tsp.
Salad dressing, mayonnaise-type, reduced-calorie	1 Tbsp.
Salad dressing (oil varieties)	1 Tbsp.

 Salad dressing, reduced-calorie	2 Tbsp.

(Two tablespoons of low-calorie salad dressing is a free food.)

SATURATED FATS

Butter	1 tsp.
★ Bacon	1 slice
Chitterlings	1/2 ounce
Coconut, shredded	2 Tbsp.
Coffee whitener, liquid	2 Tbsp.
Coffee whitener, powder	4 tsp.
Cream (light, coffee, table)	2 Tbsp.
Cream, sour	2 Tbsp.
Cream (heavy, whipping)	1 Tbsp.
Cream cheese	1 Tbsp.
★ Salt pork	1/4 ounce

400 mg or more of sodium per exchange

★ *400 mg or more of sodium if two or more exchanges are eaten*

Index